Math Related to Drug Administration

Curren

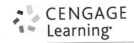

CENGAGE
Learning·

Australia • Brazil • Japan • Korea • Mexico • Singapore • Spain • United Kingdom • United States

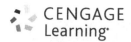
CENGAGE
Learning·

Math Related to Drug Administration

Dimensional Analysis for Meds, 4th Edition
Curren

© 2010 Delmar, Cengage Learning. All rights reserved.

Executive Editors:
Maureen Staudt
Michael Stranz

Senior Project Development Manager:
Linda deStefano

Marketing Specialist:
Courtney Sheldon

Senior Production/Manufacturing Manager:
Donna M. Brown

Production Editorial Manager:
Kim Fry

Sr. Rights Acquisition Account Manager:
Todd Osborne

For product information and technology assistance, contact us at
Cengage Learning Customer & Sales Support, 1-800-354-9706
For permission to use material from this text or product,
submit all requests online at **cengage.com/permissions**
Further permissions questions can be emailed to
permissionrequest@cengage.com

This book contains select works from existing Cengage Learning resources and was produced by Cengage Learning Custom Solutions for collegiate use. As such, those adopting and/or contributing to this work are responsible for editorial content accuracy, continuity and completeness.

Compilation © 2012 Cengage Learning
ISBN-13: 978-1-285-13040-8

ISBN-10: 1-285-13040-5

Cengage Learning
5191 Natorp Boulevard
Mason, Ohio 45040
USA
Cengage Learning is a leading provider of customized learning solutions with office locations around the globe, including Singapore, the United Kingdom, Australia, Mexico, Brazil, and Japan. Locate your local office at:
international.cengage.com/region.

Cengage Learning products are represented in Canada by Nelson Education, Ltd. For your lifelong learning solutions, visit **www.cengage.com/custom.** Visit our corporate website at **www.cengage.com.**

Printed in the United States of America

Brief Contents

1

Refresher Math

RELATIVE VALUE, ADDITION, AND SUBTRACTION OF DECIMALS

Objectives

The learner will:

1. identify the relative value of decimals.

2. add decimals.

3. subtract decimals.

Prerequisites

Recognize the abbreviations mg, for milligram, and g, for gram, as drug measures.

In the course of administering medications, you will be dealing with decimal fraction dosages on a daily basis. The first two chapters of this text provide a complete refresher on everything you need to know about decimals, including safety measures when you do calculations both manually and with a calculator. We'll start with a review of the range of decimal values you will see in dosages. This will enable you to recognize which of two or more numbers has the greater (or lesser) value—a skill you will use constantly in your professional career.

RELATIVE VALUE OF DECIMALS

The most helpful fact to remember about decimals is that **our monetary system of dollars and cents is a decimal system**. The whole numbers in dosages have the same relative value as dollars, and decimal fractions have the same value as cents: **the greater the number, the greater the value**. If you keep this in mind, you will have already learned the most important safety measure of dealing with decimals in dosages.

The range of drug dosages, which includes decimal fractions, stretches from millions on the whole number side, to thousandths on the decimal side. Refer to the decimal scale in Figure 1-1, and locate the decimal point, which

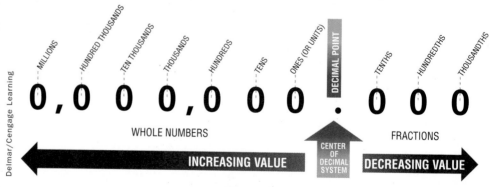

Figure 1-1

is slightly to the right on this scale. Notice the whole numbers on the left of the scale, which rise increasingly in value from ones (units) to millions, which is the largest whole-number drug dosage in current use.

The first determiner of the relative value of decimals is the presence of whole numbers. The greater the whole number, the greater the value.

EXAMPLE 1   10.1 is greater than 9.15

EXAMPLE 2   3.2 is greater than 2.99

EXAMPLE 3   7.01 is greater than 6.99

Problems 1.1

Choose the greatest value in each set.

1. a) 3.5   b) 2.7   c) 4.2   _____

2. a) 6.15   b) 5.95   c) 4.54   _____

3. a) 12.02   b) 10.19   c) 11.04   _____

4. a) 2.5   b) 1.75   c) 0.75   _____

5. a) 4.3   b) 2.75   c) 5.1   _____

6. a) 6.15   b) 7.4   c) 5.95   _____

7. a) 7.25   b) 8.1   c) 9.37   _____

8. a) 4.25   b) 5.1   c) 3.75   _____

9. a) 9.4   b) 8.75   c) 7.4   _____

10. a) 5.1   b) 6.33   c) 4.2   _____

Answers **1.** c **2.** a **3.** a **4.** a **5.** c **6.** b **7.** c **8.** b **9.** a **10.** b

If, however, the whole numbers are the same—for example, **10**.2 and **10**.7—or there are no whole numbers—for example, **0**.25 and **0**.35—**then the fraction will determine the relative value**. Let's take a closer look at the fractional side of the scale (refer to Figure 1-2).

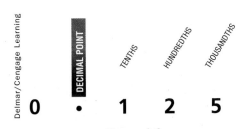

Figure 1-2

It is necessary to **consider only three figures after the decimal point on the fractional side,** because drug dosages measured as decimal fractions do not contain more than three digits; for example, 0.125 mg. Notice that a **zero is used to replace the whole number** in this decimal fraction and in all dosages that do not contain a whole number.

If a decimal fraction is not preceded by a whole number, a zero is used in front of the decimal point to emphasize that the number is a fraction.

EXAMPLE   **0.**125   **0.**1   **0.**45

Look again at Figure 1-2. The numbers to the right of the decimal point represent **tenths, hundredths,** and **thousandths,** in that order. When you see a decimal fraction in which the **whole numbers are the same,** or there are **no whole numbers,** stop and look first at the number representing **tenths.**

The fraction with the greater number representing tenths has the greater value.

EXAMPLE 1   0.3 is greater than 0.27

EXAMPLE 2   0.4 is greater than 0.29

EXAMPLE 3   1.2 is greater than 1.19

EXAMPLE 4   3.5 is greater than 3.2

Problems 1.2

Choose the greatest value in each set.

1. a) 0.4	b) 0.2	c) 0.5	_____
2. a) 2.73	b) 2.61	c) 2.87	_____
3. a) 0.19	b) 0.61	c) 0.34	_____
4. a) 3.5	b) 3.75	c) 3.25	_____
5. a) 0.3	b) 0.25	c) 0.4	_____
6. a) 1.35	b) 1.29	c) 1.4	_____
7. a) 2.5	b) 2.7	c) 2.35	_____
8. a) 4.51	b) 4.75	c) 4.8	_____
9. a) 0.8	b) 0.3	c) 0.4	_____
10. a) 2.1	b) 2.05	c) 2.15	_____

Answers   1. c.   **2.** c   **3.** b   **4.** b   **5.** c   **6.** c   **7.** b   **8.** c   **9.** a   **10.** c

If in decimal fractions the numbers representing **the tenths are identical**—for example, 0.25 and 0.27—then **the number representing the hundredths will determine the relative value.**

When the tenths are identical, the fraction with the greater number representing hundredths will have the greater value.

EXAMPLE 1   0.27 is greater than 0.25

EXAMPLE 2   0.15 is greater than 0.1 (0.1 is the same as 0.10)

Extra zeros on the end of decimal fractions are omitted in drug dosages because they can easily be misread and lead to errors.

EXAMPLE 3   2.25 is greater than 2.2 (same as 2.20)

EXAMPLE 4   9.77 is greater than 9.7 (same as 9.70)

Problems 1.3

Choose the greatest value in each set.

1.	a) 0.12	b) 0.15	c) 0.17	_____
2.	a) 1.2	b) 1.24	c) 1.23	_____
3.	a) 0.37	b) 0.3	c) 0.36	_____
4.	a) 3.27	b) 3.25	c) 3.21	_____
5.	a) 0.16	b) 0.11	c) 0.19	_____
6.	a) 4.23	b) 4.2	c) 4.09	_____
7.	a) 3.27	b) 3.21	c) 3.29	_____
8.	a) 2.75	b) 2.73	c) 2.78	_____
9.	a) 0.31	b) 0.37	c) 0.33	_____
10.	a) 0.43	b) 0.45	c) 0.44	_____

Answers   **1.** c   **2.** b   **3.** a   **4.** a   **5.** c   **6.** a   **7.** c   **8.** c   **9.** b   **10.** b

Problems 1.4

Which fraction has the greater value?

   a) 0.125   b) 0.25

Answer   If you chose 0.125, you have just made a serious drug dosage error. Look again at the numbers representing the tenths, and you will see that 0.**25** is greater than 0.**1**25. Remember that extra zeros are omitted in decimal fraction dosages because they can lead to errors. In this fraction, 0.25 is the same as 0.250, which is exactly double the value of 0.125. **Check the tenths carefully, regardless of the total of numbers after the decimal point.**

EXAMPLE 1	0.15 (same as 0.150) is greater than 0.125
EXAMPLE 2	0.3 (same as 0.30) is greater than 0.15
EXAMPLE 3	0.75 (same as 0.750) is greater than 0.325
EXAMPLE 4	0.8 (same as 0.80) is greater than 0.16

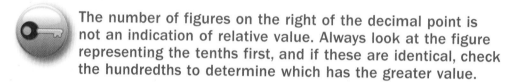

The number of figures on the right of the decimal point is not an indication of relative value. Always look at the figure representing the tenths first, and if these are identical, check the hundredths to determine which has the greater value.

This completes your introduction to the relative value of decimals. The key points just reviewed will cover all situations in dosage calculations in which you will have to recognize greater and lesser values. Test yourself more extensively on this information in the following problems.

Problems 1.5

Choose the greatest value in each set.

1. a) 0.24	b) 0.5	c) 0.125	_____
2. a) 0.4	b) 0.45	c) 0.5	_____
3. a) 7.5	b) 6.25	c) 4.75	_____
4. a) 0.3	b) 0.25	c) 0.35	_____
5. a) 1.125	b) 1.75	c) 1.5	_____
6. a) 4.5	b) 4.75	c) 4.25	_____
7. a) 0.1	b) 0.01	c) 0.04	_____
8. a) 5.75	b) 6.25	c) 6.5	_____
9. a) 0.6	b) 0.16	c) 0.06	_____
10. a) 3.55	b) 2.95	c) 3.7	_____

Answers   1. b   **2.** c   **3.** a   **4.** c   **5.** b   **6.** b   **7.** a   **8.** c   **9.** a   **10.** c

ADDITION AND SUBTRACTION OF DECIMALS

Complex addition and subtraction of decimals should be done with a calculator, but, on occasion, time can be saved by doing simple calculations without one. Let's start by looking at a few key points that will make manual solution safer.

 When you write down the numbers, line up the decimal points.

EXAMPLE   To add 0.25 and 0.27

    0.25   0.25
   +0.27 is safe   +0.27 is unsafe; it could lead to errors.

 Always add or subtract from right to left.

If you decide to write down the numbers, **do not confuse yourself by trying to "eyeball" the answer**. Also, write any numbers carried or rewrite those reduced by borrowing if you find this helpful.

EXAMPLE 1   When adding 0.25 and 0.27

       1
      0.25
    +0.27   Add the 5 and 7 first, then the 2, 2, and
      0.52   the 1 you carried; work from right to left

EXAMPLE 2   When subtracting 0.63 from 0.71

       61
      0.71   Borrow 1 from 7 and rewrite as 6
    −0.63   Write the borrowed 1; subtract 3 from 11
      0.08   Subtract 6 from 6; work from right to left

 Add zeros as necessary to make the fractions of equal length.

Adding zeros to make the fractions of equal length does not alter the value of the fractions, and it helps prevent confusion and mistakes.

EXAMPLE   When subtracting 0.125 from 0.25

    0.25   0.250
    0.125   becomes   0.125   Answer = **0.125**

If you follow these simple rules and make them a habit, you will automatically reduce calculation errors. The problems on the following page will give you an excellent opportunity to practice addition and subtraction.

Problems 1.6

Add decimals.

1. $0.25 + 0.55$ = _____

2. $0.1 + 2.25$ = _____

3. $1.74 + 0.76$ = _____

4. $1.4 + 0.02$ = _____

5. $2.3 + 1.45$ = _____

6. $3.75 + 1.05$ = _____

7. $6.35 + 2.05$ = _____

8. $5.57 + 4.03$ = _____

9. $0.33 + 2.42$ = _____

10. $1.44 + 3.06$ = _____

Subtract decimals.

11. $1.25 - 1.125$ = _____

12. $3.25 - 0.65$ = _____

13. $2.3 - 1.45$ = _____

14. $0.02 - 0.01$ = _____

15. $5.5 - 2.5$ = _____

16. $7.33 - 4.03$ = _____

17. $4.25 - 1.75$ = _____

18. $0.07 - 0.035$ = _____

19. $0.235 - 0.12$ = _____

20. $5.75 - 0.95$ = _____

Answers 1. 0.8 **2.** 2.35 **3.** 2.5 **4.** 1.42 **5.** 3.75 **6.** 4.8 **7.** 8.4 **8.** 9.6 **9.** 2.75 **10.** 4.5
11. 0.125 **12.** 2.6 **13.** 0.85 **14.** 0.01 **15.** 3 **16.** 3.3 **17.** 2.5 **18.** 0.035 **19.** 0.115 **20.** 4.8
Note: If you did not add a zero before the decimal point in answers that do not contain a whole number, or failed to eliminate unnecessary zeros from the end of decimal fractions, your answers are incorrect.

Summary

This concludes the refresher on relative value, addition, and subtraction of simple decimal fractions. The important points to remember from this chapter are:

- If a decimal fraction contains a whole number, the value of the whole number is the first determiner of relative value.

- If a fraction does not include a whole number, a zero is placed in front of the decimal point to emphasize that it is a fractional dosage.

- If there is no whole number, or if the whole numbers are the same, the number representing the tenths in the decimal fraction will be the next determiner of relative value.

- If the tenths in decimal fractions are identical, the number representing hundredths will determine relative value.

- When manually adding or subtracting decimal fractions, first line up the decimal points, then add or subtract from right to left.

- Extra zeros on the end of decimal fractions can be a source of error in drug dosages, and are routinely eliminated.

Summary Self-Test

Choose the decimal with the greatest value.

1. a) 2.45   b) 2.57   c) 2.19   _____
2. a) 3.07   b) 3.17   c) 3.71   _____
3. a) 0.12   b) 0.02   c) 0.01   _____
4. a) 5.31   b) 5.35   c) 6.01   _____
5. a) 4.5   b) 4.51   c) 4.15   _____
6. a) 0.015   b) 0.15   c) 0.1   _____
7. a) 1.3   b) 1.25   c) 1.35   _____
8. a) 0.1   b) 0.2   c) 0.25   _____
9. a) 0.125   b) 0.1   c) 0.05   _____
10. a) 13.7   b) 13.5   c) 13.25   _____

11. If you have medication tablets whose strength is 0.1 mg and you must give 0.3 mg, you will need

    a) 1 tablet.   b) less than 1 tablet.   c) more than 1 tablet.   _____

12. If you have tablets with a strength of 0.25 mg and you must give 0.125 mg, you will need

    a) 1 tablet.   b) less than 1 tablet.   c) more than 1 tablet.   _____

13. If you have an order to give a dosage of 7.5 mg and the tablets have a strength of 3.75 mg, you will need

    a) 1 tablet.   b) less than 1 tablet.   c) more than 1 tablet.   _____

14. If the order is to give 0.5 mg and the tablet strength is 0.5 mg, you will give

    a) 1 tablet.   b) less than 1 tablet.   c) more than 1 tablet.   _____

15. The order is to give 0.5 mg and the tablets have a strength of 0.25 mg. You must give

    a) 1 tablet.   b) less than 1 tablet.   c) more than 1 tablet.   _____

Add the decimals manually.

16. $1.31 + 0.4$ = _____   20. $1.3 + 1.04$ = _____
17. $0.15 + 0.25$ = _____   21. $4.7 + 3.03$ = _____
18. $2.5 + 0.75$ = _____   22. $0.5 + 0.5$ = _____
19. $3.2 + 2.17$ = _____   23. $5.4 + 2.6$ = _____

24. You have just given two tablets with a dosage strength of 3.5 mg each. What was the total dosage administered?   _____

25. You are to give your patient one tablet labeled 0.5 mg and one labeled 0.25 mg. What is the total dosage of these two tablets?   _____

26. If you give two tablets labeled 0.02 mg, what total dosage will you administer?   _____

27. You are to give one tablet labeled 0.8 mg and two tablets labeled 0.4 mg. What is the total dosage? _____

28. You have two tablets: one is labeled 0.15 mg and the other 0.3 mg. What is the total dosage of these two tablets? _____

Subtract the decimals manually.

29. $4.32 - 3.1$ = _____

30. $2.1 - 1.91$ = _____

31. $3.73 - 1.93$ = _____

32. $5.75 - 4.05$ = _____

33. $1.3 - 0.02$ = _____

34. $0.2 - 0.07$ = _____

35. $3.95 - 0.35$ = _____

36. $1.9 - 0.08$ = _____

37. Your patient is to receive a dosage of 7.5 mg and you have only one tablet labeled 3.75 mg. How many more milligrams must you give? _____

38. You have a tablet labeled 0.02 mg and your patient is to receive 0.06 mg. How many more milligrams must you give? _____

39. The tablet available is labeled 0.5 mg, but you must give a dosage of 1.5 mg. How many more milligrams will you need to obtain the correct dosage? _____

40. Your patient is to receive a dosage of 1.2 mg and you have one tablet labeled 0.6 mg. What additional dosage in milligrams will you need? _____

41. You must give your patient a dosage of 2.2 mg, but you have only two tablets labeled 0.55 mg. What additional dosage in milligrams will you need? _____

Determine how many tablets will be needed to give the dosages.

42. Tablets are labeled 0.01 mg. You must give 0.02 mg. _____

43. Tablets are labeled 2.5 mg. You must give 5 mg. _____

44. Tablets are labeled 0.25 mg. Give 0.125 mg. _____

45. Tablets are 0.5 mg. Give 1.5 mg. _____

46. A dosage of 1.8 mg is ordered. Tablets are 0.6 mg. _____

47. Tablets available are 0.04 mg. You are to give 0.02 mg. _____

48. The dosage ordered is 3.5 mg. The tablets available are 1.75 mg. _____

49. Prepare a dosage of 3.2 mg using tablets with a strength of 1.6 mg. _____

50. You have tablets labeled 0.25 mg and a dosage of 0.375 mg is ordered. _____

Answers	11. c	22. 1	33. 1.28	44. ½ tab
1. b	12. b	23. 8	34. 0.13	45. 3 tab
2. c	13. c	24. 7 mg	35. 3.6	46. 3 tab
3. a	14. a	25. 0.75 mg	36. 1.82	47. ½ tab
4. c	15. c	26. 0.04 mg	37. 3.75 mg	48. 2 tab
5. b	16. 1.71	27. 1.6 mg	38. 0.04 mg	49. 2 tab
6. b	17. 0.4	28. 0.45 mg	39. 1 mg	50. 1½ tab
7. c	18. 3.25	29. 1.22	40. 0.6 mg	
8. c	19. 5.37	30. 0.19	41. 1.1 mg	
9. a	20. 2.34	31. 1.8	42. 2 tab	
10. a	21. 7.73	32. 1.7	43. 2 tab	

Note: If you did not add a zero before the decimal point in answers that did not contain a whole number, or failed to eliminate unnecessary zeros from the end of decimal fractions, your answers are incorrect.

MULTIPLICATION AND DIVISION OF DECIMALS

Multiplication and division are integral parts of dosage calculations. As is the case with addition and subtraction, some multiplication and division problems involving dosages can be done manually, so the basic steps in multiplication and division are reviewed in this chapter. In addition, a number of shortcuts will be introduced that can make numbers easier to work with, especially those containing decimal fractions. And for those calculations that are more safely handled with a calculator, safety in calculator use will be discussed.

MULTIPLICATION OF DECIMALS

The main precaution in multiplication of decimals is the **placement of the decimal point in the answer**, which is called the **product**.

> The decimal point in the product of decimal fractions is placed the same number of places to the left in the product as the total of numbers following the decimal points in the fractions multiplied.

EXAMPLE 1   Multiply 0.35 by 0.5

It is safer to begin by lining up the numbers to be multiplied on the right side. Then, disregard the decimals during multiplication.

$$\begin{array}{r} 0.35 \\ \times\ \ 0.5 \\ \hline 175 \end{array}$$

The product/answer is 175; 0.35 has two numbers after the decimal and 0.5 has one. Place the decimal point three places to the left in the product to make it .175, then add a zero (0) in front of the decimal to emphasize the fraction.

Answer = **0.175**

Objectives

The learner will:

1. define product, numerator, and denominator.
2. multiply decimal fractions.
3. divide decimal fractions.
4. simplify common fractions containing decimal numbers.
5. reduce fractions using common denominators.
6. reduce common fractions that end in zeros.
7. express answers to the nearest tenth and hundredth.
8. use a calculator to multiply and divide.

Prerequisite

Chapter 1

EXAMPLE 2   Multiply 1.61 by 0.2

$$\begin{array}{r} 1.61 \\ \times\ \underline{\ 0.2} \\ 322 \end{array}$$ Line up the numbers on the right

The product is 322; 1.61 has two numbers after the decimal point and 0.2 has one. Place the decimal point three places to the left in the product so that 322 becomes .322, then add a zero in front of the decimal to emphasize the fraction.

Answer = **0.322**

If the product contains insufficient numbers for correct placement of the decimal point, add as many zeros as necessary to the left of the product to correct this.

EXAMPLE 3   Multiply 1.5 by 0.06

$$\begin{array}{r} 1.5 \\ \times\ \underline{0.06} \\ 90 \end{array}$$ Line up the numbers on the right

The product is 90; 1.5 has one number after the decimal point and 0.06 has two. To place the decimal three places to the left in the product, a zero must be added, making it .090. Eliminate the excess zero from the end of the fraction, and add a zero in front of the decimal point.

Answer = **0.09**

EXAMPLE 4   Multiply 0.21 by 0.32

$$\begin{array}{r} 0.21 \\ \times\ \underline{0.32} \\ 42 \\ \underline{63\ \ } \\ 672 \end{array}$$

42
63   Indent second number multiplication
672   Add the totals

In this example, 0.21 has two numbers after the decimal point and 0.32 also has two. Add a zero in front of 672 to allow correct placement of the decimal point, making it .0672, then add a zero in front of the fraction to emphasize it.

Answer = **0.0672**

EXAMPLE 5   Multiply 0.12 by 0.2

$$\begin{array}{r} 0.12 \\ \times\ \underline{\ 0.2} \\ 24 \end{array}$$

In this example, there are a total of three numbers after the decimal points in 0.12 and 0.2. Add a zero in front of 24 for correct decimal placement, making it .024, then add a zero in front of .024 to emphasize the fraction.

Answer = **0.024**

Problems 2.1

Multiply the decimal fractions without using a calculator.

1. 0.45×0.2 = _____

2. 0.35×0.12 = _____

3. 1.3×0.05 = _____

4. 0.7×0.04 = _____

5. 0.4×0.17 = _____

6. 2.14×0.03 = _____

7. 1.4×0.4 = _____

8. 3.3×1.2 = _____

9. 2.7×2.2 = _____

10. 2.1×0.3 = _____

Answers **1.** 0.09 **2.** 0.042 **3.** 0.065 **4.** 0.028 **5.** 0.068 **6.** 0.0642 **7.** 0.56 **8.** 3.96 **9.** 5.94 **10.** 0.63

DIVISION OF DECIMAL FRACTIONS

A calculator may also be used for division of complex decimal fractions. However, let's start by reviewing the terminology of common fraction division, and **three important precalculator** steps that may make final manual division easier: **elimination of decimal points, reduction of the fractions,** and **reduction of numbers ending in zero**. The following is a sample of a common fraction division seen in dosages.

EXAMPLE 1 $\dfrac{0.25}{0.125} = \dfrac{\text{numerator}}{\text{denominator}}$

You'll recall that the **top number** in a common fraction is called the **numerator**, whereas the **bottom number** is called the **denominator**. If you have trouble remembering which is which, think of **D**, for **down**, for **denominator**. The denominator is on the bottom. With this basic terminology reviewed, we are now ready to look at preliminary math steps that can be used to simplify a fraction or actually solve an equation and eliminate the need for calculator division.

ELIMINATION OF DECIMAL POINTS

Decimal points can be eliminated from numbers in a decimal fraction without changing its value, if they are moved the same number of places in one numerator and one denominator.

To eliminate the decimal points from decimal fractions, move them the same number of places to the right in a numerator and a denominator until they are eliminated from both. Zeros may have to be added to accomplish this.

EXAMPLE 1 $\dfrac{0.25}{0.125}$ becomes $\dfrac{250}{125}$

The decimal point must be moved three places to the right in the denominator 0.125 to make it 125. Therefore, it must be moved three places to the right in the numerator 0.25, which requires the addition of one zero to make it 250.

EXAMPLE 2 $\dfrac{0.3}{0.15}$ becomes $\dfrac{30}{15}$

The decimal point must be moved two places in 0.15 to make it 15, so it must be moved two places in 0.3, which requires the addition of one zero to become 30.

EXAMPLE 3 $\dfrac{1.5}{2}$ becomes $\dfrac{15}{20}$

Move the decimal point one place in 1.5 to make it 15; add one zero to 2 to make it 20.

EXAMPLE 4 $\dfrac{4.5}{0.95}$ becomes $\dfrac{450}{95}$

 Eliminating the decimal points from a decimal fraction before final division does not alter the value of the fraction, or the answer obtained in the final division.

Problems 2.2

Eliminate the decimal points from these common fractions.

1. $\dfrac{17.5}{2}$ = _____

2. $\dfrac{0.5}{25}$ = _____

3. $\dfrac{6.3}{0.6}$ = _____

4. $\dfrac{3.76}{0.4}$ = _____

5. $\dfrac{8.4}{0.7}$ = _____

6. $\dfrac{0.1}{0.05}$ = _____

7. $\dfrac{0.9}{0.03}$ = _____

8. $\dfrac{10.75}{2.5}$ = _____

9. $\dfrac{0.4}{0.04}$ = _____

10. $\dfrac{1.2}{0.4}$ = _____

Answers 1. $\dfrac{175}{20}$ 2. $\dfrac{5}{250}$ 3. $\dfrac{63}{6}$ 4. $\dfrac{376}{40}$ 5. $\dfrac{84}{7}$ 6. $\dfrac{10}{5}$ 7. $\dfrac{90}{3}$ 8. $\dfrac{1075}{250}$ 9. $\dfrac{40}{4}$ 10. $\dfrac{12}{4}$

REDUCTION OF FRACTIONS

Once the decimal points are eliminated, a second simplification step is to reduce the numbers as far as possible using common denominators/divisors, the largest number that will divide both a numerator and a denominator.

 To further reduce fractions, divide numbers by their greatest common denominator (the largest number that will divide into both a numerator and a denominator).

The **greatest common denominator** is usually **2, 3, 4, 5, or multiples of these numbers**, such as 6, 8, 25, and so on.

EXAMPLE 1 $\dfrac{175}{20}$ The greatest common denominator is 5

$$\dfrac{\cancel{175}}{\cancel{20}} = \dfrac{35}{4}$$

EXAMPLE 2 $\dfrac{63}{6}$ The greatest common denominator is 3

$$\dfrac{\cancel{63}}{\cancel{6}} = \dfrac{21}{2}$$

EXAMPLE 3 $\dfrac{1075}{250}$ The greatest common denominator is 25

$$\dfrac{\cancel{1075}}{\cancel{250}} = \dfrac{43}{10}$$

There is a second way you could have reduced the fraction in Example 3, and it is equally as correct. Divide by 5, then by 5 again.

$$\dfrac{\cancel{1075}}{\cancel{250}} = \dfrac{\cancel{215}}{\cancel{50}} = \dfrac{43}{10}$$

If the greatest common denominator is difficult to determine, reduce several times by using smaller common denominators.

EXAMPLE 4 $\dfrac{376}{40} = \dfrac{47}{5}$ Divide by 8

Or divide by 4, then 2 $\dfrac{\cancel{376}}{\cancel{40}} = \dfrac{\cancel{94}}{\cancel{10}} = \dfrac{47}{5}$

Or divide by 2, then 2, then 2 $\dfrac{\cancel{376}}{\cancel{40}} = \dfrac{\cancel{188}}{\cancel{20}} = \dfrac{\cancel{94}}{\cancel{10}} = \dfrac{47}{5}$

Remember that **simple numbers are easiest to work with**, and the time spent in extra reductions may be well worth the payoff in safety.

Problems 2.3

Reduce the fractions in preparation for final division.

1. $\dfrac{84}{8}$ = _____

2. $\dfrac{20}{16}$ = _____

3. $\dfrac{250}{325}$ = _____

4. $\dfrac{96}{34}$ = _____

5. $\dfrac{175}{20}$ = _____

6. $\dfrac{40}{14}$ = _____

7. $\dfrac{82}{28}$ = _____   9. $\dfrac{50}{75}$ = _____

8. $\dfrac{100}{75}$ = _____   10. $\dfrac{60}{88}$ = _____

Answers 1. $\dfrac{21}{2}$ 2. $\dfrac{5}{4}$ 3. $\dfrac{10}{13}$ 4. $\dfrac{48}{17}$ 5. $\dfrac{35}{4}$ 6. $\dfrac{20}{7}$ 7. $\dfrac{41}{14}$ 8. $\dfrac{4}{3}$ 9. $\dfrac{2}{3}$ 10. $\dfrac{15}{22}$

REDUCTION OF NUMBERS ENDING IN ZERO

The third type of simplification is not solely related to decimal fractions but is best covered at this time. This concerns reductions in a common fraction when both a numerator and a denominator end with zeros.

Numbers that end in a zero or zeros may be reduced by crossing off the same number of zeros in both a numerator and a denominator.

EXAMPLE 1 $\dfrac{800}{250}$

In this fraction, the numerator, 800, has two zeros, but the denominator, 250, has one zero. The number of zeros crossed off must be the same in both numerator and denominator, so only one zero can be eliminated from each.

$$\dfrac{80\cancel{0}}{25\cancel{0}} = \dfrac{80}{25} \qquad \text{Reduce by } 5 = \dfrac{16}{5}$$

EXAMPLE 2 $\dfrac{24\cancel{00}}{20\cancel{00}} = \dfrac{24}{20}$ Reduce by $4 = \dfrac{6}{5}$

Two zeros can be eliminated from the denominator and the numerator in this fraction.

EXAMPLE 3 $\dfrac{15\cancel{000}}{30\cancel{000}} = \dfrac{15}{30}$ Reduce by $15 = \dfrac{1}{2}$

In this fraction, three zeros can be eliminated.

Problems 2.4

Reduce the fractions to their lowest terms.

1. $\dfrac{50}{250}$ = _____   4. $\dfrac{1,000,000}{750,000}$ = _____

2. $\dfrac{120}{50}$ = _____   5. $\dfrac{800}{150}$ = _____

3. $\dfrac{2500}{1500}$ = _____   6. $\dfrac{110}{100}$ = _____

7. $\dfrac{200,000}{150,000}$ = _____

9. $\dfrac{60}{40}$ = _____

8. $\dfrac{1000}{800}$ = _____

10. $\dfrac{150}{200}$ = _____

Answers   1. $\frac{1}{5}$ **2.** $\frac{12}{5}$ **3.** $\frac{5}{3}$ **4.** $\frac{4}{3}$ **5.** $\frac{16}{3}$ **6.** $\frac{11}{10}$ **7.** $\frac{4}{3}$ **8.** $\frac{5}{4}$ **9.** $\frac{3}{2}$ **10.** $\frac{3}{4}$

USING A CALCULATOR

Calculators vary in how addition, subtraction, division, and multiplication must be entered, and in the number of fractional numbers displayed after the decimal point. The first precaution in calculator use is to ensure you **know how to use the one available to you.** If you must do frequent calculations, it would be wise to buy and use your own. The next precaution—and this is critical—is to enter decimal numbers correctly, which includes **entering the decimal points**. This is not as easy to remember as it sounds, and this is a step where dosage calculation errors can occur.

Calculator entry errors tend to be repetitive, so visually check each entry before entering the next.

EXPRESSING TO THE NEAREST TENTH

When a fraction is reduced as much as possible, it is ready for final division. If necessary, this is done using a calculator to **divide the numerator by the denominator**. Dosage answers are most frequently rounded off and expressed as decimal fractions to the nearest tenth.

To express an answer to the nearest tenth, the division is carried to hundredths (two places after the decimal). When the number representing hundredths is 5 or larger, the number representing tenths is increased by one.

EXAMPLE 1 $\dfrac{0.35}{0.4} = 0.35 \div 0.4 = 0.87$

Answer = **0.9**

The number representing hundredths is 7, so the number representing tenths is increased by one: 0.87 becomes 0.9.

EXAMPLE 2 $\dfrac{0.5}{0.3} = 0.5 \div 0.3 = 1.66 = \textbf{1.7}$

The number representing hundredths, 6, is larger than 5, so 1.66 becomes 1.7.

EXAMPLE 3 $\dfrac{0.16}{0.3} = 0.53 = \textbf{0.5}$

The number representing hundredths, 3, is less than 5, so the number representing tenths, 5, remains unchanged.

EXAMPLE 4 $\frac{0.2}{0.3} = 0.66 = \mathbf{0.7}$

EXAMPLE 5   An answer of 1.42 remains **1.4**.

EXAMPLE 6   An answer of 1.86 becomes **1.9**.

Problems 2.5

Use a calculator to divide the common fractions. Express answers to the nearest tenth.

1. $\frac{5.1}{2.3}$ = _____

2. $\frac{0.9}{0.7}$ = _____

3. $\frac{3.7}{2}$ = _____

4. $\frac{6}{1.3}$ = _____

5. $\frac{1.5}{2.1}$ = _____

6. $\frac{2.7}{1.1}$ = _____

7. $\frac{4.2}{5}$ = _____

8. $\frac{0.5}{2.5}$ = _____

9. $\frac{5.2}{0.91}$ = _____

10. $\frac{2.4}{2.7}$ = _____

Answers   1. 2.2   **2.** 1.3   **3.** 1.9   **4.** 4.6   **5.** 0.7   **6.** 2.5   **7.** 0.8   **8.** 0.2   **9.** 5.7   **10.** 0.9

EXPRESSING TO THE NEAREST HUNDREDTH

Some drugs are administered in dosages carried to the nearest hundredth. This is common in pediatric dosages, and in drugs that alter a vital function of the body, for example, heart rate.

   To express an answer to the nearest hundredth, the division is carried to thousandths (three places after the decimal point). When the number representing thousandths is 5 or larger, the number representing hundredths is increased by one.

EXAMPLE 1   0.736   becomes   **0.74**

The number representing thousandths, 6, is larger than 5, so the number representing hundredths, 3, is increased by one to become 4.

EXAMPLE 2   0.777   becomes   **0.78**

EXAMPLE 3   0.373   remains   **0.37**

The number representing thousandths, 3, is less than 5, so the number representing hundredths, 7, remains unchanged.

EXAMPLE 4   0.934   remains   **0.93**

Problems 2.6

Express the numbers to the nearest hundredth.

1. 0.175 = _____

2. 0.344 = _____

3. 1.853 = _____

4. 0.306 = _____

5. 3.015 = _____

6. 2.154 = _____

7. 1.081 = _____

8. 1.327 = _____

9. 0.739 = _____

10. 0.733 = _____

11. 2.072 = _____

12 0.089 = _____

Answers 1. 0.18 **2.** 0.34 **3.** 1.85 **4.** 0.31 **5.** 3.02 **6.** 2.15 **7.** 1.08 **8.** 1.33 **9.** 0.74
10. 0.73 **11.** 2.07 **12.** 0.09

Summary

This concludes the chapter on multiplication and division of decimals. The important points to remember from this chapter are:

- When decimal fractions are multiplied manually, the decimal point is placed the same number of places to the left in the product as the total of numbers after the decimal points in the fractions multiplied.

- Zeros must be placed in front of a product if it contains insufficient numbers for the correct placement of the decimal point.

- Excess trailing zeros are eliminated in dosages.

- To simplify fractions for final division, the preliminary steps of eliminating decimal points, reducing the numbers by common denominators, and reducing numbers ending in zeros can be used.

- To express to tenths, increase the answer by one if the number representing the thousandths is 5 or larger.

- To express to hundredths, increase the answer by one if the number representing the thousandths is 5 or larger.

- Practice using a calculator until proficiency is achieved.

- All calculator entries and answers must be double-checked.

- Calculator running totals should be disregarded because they can cause confusion.

- A personal calculator is a must if frequent calculations are necessary.

Summary Self-Test

Multiply the decimals. A calculator may be used.

1. 1.49×0.05 = _____
2. 0.15×3.04 = _____
3. 0.025×3.5 = _____
4. 0.55×2.5 = _____
5. 1.31×2.07 = _____

6. 5.3×1.02 = _____
7. 0.35×1.25 = _____
8. 4.32×0.05 = _____
9. 0.2×0.02 = _____
10. 0.4×1.75 = _____

11. You are to administer four tablets with a dosage strength of 0.04 mg each. What total dosage are you giving? _____

12. You have given 2½ (2.5) tablets with a strength of 1.25 mg per tablet. What total dosage is this? _____

13. The tablets your patient is to receive are labeled 0.1 mg, and you are to give 3½ (3.5) tablets. What total dosage is this? _____

14. You gave your patient 3 tablets labeled 0.75 mg each, and he was to receive a total of 2.25 mg. Did he receive the correct dosage? _____

15. The tablets available for your patient are labeled 12.5 mg, and you are to give 4½ (4.5) tablets. What total dosage will this be? _____

16. Your patient is to receive a dosage of 4.5 mg. The tablets available are labeled 3.5 mg, and there are 2½ tablets in his medication drawer. Is this a correct dosage? _____

Divide the fractions. Express answers to the nearest tenth. A calculator may be used.

17. $\dfrac{1.3}{0.7}$ = _____
18. $\dfrac{1.9}{3.2}$ = _____
19. $\dfrac{32.5}{9}$ = _____
20. $\dfrac{0.04}{0.1}$ = _____
21. $\dfrac{1.45}{1.2}$ = _____
22. $\dfrac{250}{1000}$ = _____
23. $\dfrac{0.8}{0.09}$ = _____

24. $\dfrac{2,000,000}{1,500,000}$ = _____
25. $\dfrac{4.1}{2.05}$ = _____
26. $\dfrac{7.3}{12}$ = _____
27. $\dfrac{150,000}{120,000}$ = _____
28. $\dfrac{0.15}{0.08}$ = _____
29. $\dfrac{2700}{900}$ = _____
30. $\dfrac{0.25}{0.15}$ = _____

Divide the fractions. Express answers to the nearest hundredth. A calculator may be used.

31. $\dfrac{900}{1700}$ = _____

32. $\dfrac{0.125}{0.3}$ = _____

33. $\dfrac{1450}{1500}$ = _____

34. $\dfrac{65}{175}$ = _____

35. $\dfrac{0.6}{1.35}$ = _____

36. $\dfrac{0.04}{0.12}$ = _____

37. $\dfrac{750}{10,000}$ = _____

38. $\dfrac{0.65}{0.8}$ = _____

39. $\dfrac{3.01}{4.2}$ = _____

40. $\dfrac{4.5}{6.1}$ = _____

41. $\dfrac{0.13}{0.25}$ = _____

42. $\dfrac{0.25}{0.7}$ = _____

43. $\dfrac{3.3}{5.1}$ = _____

44. $\dfrac{0.19}{0.7}$ = _____

45. $\dfrac{1.1}{1.3}$ = _____

46. $\dfrac{3}{4.1}$ = _____

47. $\dfrac{62}{240}$ = _____

48. $\dfrac{280,000}{300,000}$ = _____

49. $\dfrac{115}{255}$ = _____

50. $\dfrac{10}{14.3}$ = _____

Answers				
1. 0.0745	**11.** 0.16 mg	**22.** 0.3	**33.** 0.97	**44.** 0.27
2. 0.456	**12.** 3.125 mg	**23.** 8.9	**34.** 0.37	**45.** 0.85
3. 0.0875	**13.** 0.35 mg	**24.** 1.3	**35.** 0.44	**46.** 0.73
4. 1.375	**14.** Yes	**25.** 2	**36.** 0.33	**47.** 0.26
5. 2.7117	**15.** 56.25 mg	**26.** 0.6	**37.** 0.08	**48.** 0.93
6. 5.406	**16.** No	**27.** 1.3	**38.** 0.81	**49.** 0.45
7. 0.4375	**17.** 1.9	**28.** 1.9	**39.** 0.72	**50.** 0.7
8. 0.216	**18.** 0.6	**29.** 3	**40.** 0.74	
9. 0.004	**19.** 3.6	**30.** 1.7	**41.** 0.52	
10. 0.7	**20.** 0.4	**31.** 0.53	**42.** 0.36	
	21. 1.2	**32.** 0.42	**43.** 0.65	

3

SOLVING COMMON FRACTION EQUATIONS

Objectives

The learner will solve equations containing:

1. whole numbers.

2. decimal numbers.

3. multiple numbers.

Prerequisites

Chapters 1 and 2

The majority of clinical drug dosage calculations involve solving an equation containing one to five common fractions. Two examples are:

$$\frac{2}{5} \times \frac{3}{4} \quad \text{and} \quad \frac{20}{1} \times \frac{1000}{60,000} \times \frac{1200}{1} \times \frac{1}{60}$$

Two options are available to solve common fraction equations: calculator use throughout, or initial fraction reduction followed by calculator use for final division. Both options are presented in this chapter, and you may use whichever you wish, or whichever your instructor requires.

 Common fraction equations are solved by dividing the numerators by the denominators.

It is important that you do the calculations for each example and then compare them with the math provided. Just reading the examples will not teach you the calculation skills you need. The examples and problems provided incorporate all the content covered in the first two chapters. They represent the full range of calculations you will be doing on a continuing basis.

 Calculator solution of equations is most safely done by concentrating only on the entries being made, not the numbers that register and change throughout the calculation.

WHOLE-NUMBER EQUATIONS

EXAMPLE 1 **Option 1: Calculator Use Throughout**

$$\frac{2}{5} \times \frac{3}{4}$$

$2 \times 3 \div 5 \div 4$ 　　　Multiply the numerators, 2 and 3, and then divide by the denominators, 5 then 4, in continuous entries

$= 0.3$

Answer $= $ **0.3 (tenth)**

Option 2: Initial Reduction of Fractions

$$\frac{2}{5} \times \frac{3}{4}$$

$$\overset{1}{\frac{2}{5}} \times \frac{3}{\underset{2}{4}}$$ Divide the numerator, 2, and the denominator, 4, by 2
(to become 1 and 2)

$$3 \div 5 \div 2$$ Use the calculator to divide the remaining numerator, 3,
by the remaining denominators, 5 and 2

$$= 0.3$$

Answer $= $ **0.3 (tenth)**

Initial reduction of fractions in an equation can simplify final calculator entries, especially if the numbers are large, or contain decimal fractions or zeros.

EXAMPLE 2

Option 1: Calculator Use Throughout

$$\frac{250}{175} \times \frac{150}{325}$$

$$250 \times 150 \div 175 \div 325$$ Multiply the numerators, 250 and 150,
then divide by the denominators, 175
and 325

$$= 0.659$$

Answer $= $ **0.7 (tenth)** or **0.66 (hundredth)**

Option 2: Initial Reduction of Fractions

$$\frac{250}{175} \times \frac{150}{325}$$

$$\overset{10}{\underset{7}{\frac{250}{175}}} \times \overset{6}{\underset{13}{\frac{150}{325}}}$$ Divide the numerator, 250, and the denominator,
175, by 25 (to become 10 and 7); divide the
numerator, 150, and denominator, 325, by 25
(to become 6 and 13)

$$10 \times 6 \div 7 \div 13$$ Use the calculator to multiply the numerators,
10 and 6, then divide by the denominators,
7 and 13

$$= 0.659$$

Answer $= $ **0.7 (tenth)** or **0.66 (hundredth)**

EXAMPLE 3

Option 1: Calculator Use Throughout

$$\frac{7}{50} \times \frac{25}{3} \times \frac{120}{32}$$

$7 \times 25 \times 120 \div 50 \div 3 \div 32$ Multiply the numerators, 7, 25, and 120, then divide by the denominators, 50, 3, and 32

$= 4.375$

Answer $= $ **4.4 (tenth)** or **4.38 (hundredth)**

Option 2: Initial Reduction of Fractions

$$\frac{7}{50} \times \frac{25}{3} \times \frac{120}{32}$$

$$\frac{7}{\overset{}{\underset{2}{50}}} \times \frac{\overset{1}{\cancel{25}}}{3} \times \frac{\overset{15}{\cancel{120}}}{\underset{4}{\cancel{32}}}$$ Divide 25 and 50 by 25, then divide 120 and 32 by 8

$7 \times 15 \div 2 \div 3 \div 4$

$= 4.375$

Answer $= $ **4.4 (tenth)** or **4.38 (hundredth)**

EXAMPLE 4

Option 1: Calculator Use Throughout

$$\frac{20}{1} \times \frac{1000}{60,000} \times \frac{1200}{1} \times \frac{1}{60}$$

$20 \times 1000 \times 1200 \div 60,000 \div 60$

$= 6.666$

Answer $= $ **6.7 (tenth)** or **6.67 (hundredth)**

Option 2: Initial Reduction of Fractions

$$\frac{20}{1} \times \frac{1000}{60,000} \times \frac{1200}{1} \times \frac{1}{60}$$

$$\frac{\overset{1}{\cancel{20}}}{1} \times \frac{\overset{1}{\cancel{1000}}}{\underset{3}{\cancel{60,000}}} \times \frac{\overset{20}{\cancel{1200}}}{1} \times \frac{1}{\underset{1}{\cancel{60}}}$$

$20 \div 3$

$= 6.666$

Answer $= $ **6.7 (tenth)** or **6.67 (hundredth)**

EXAMPLE 5

Option 1: Calculator Use Throughout

$$\frac{2000}{1500} \times \frac{2500}{3000}$$

$2000 \times 2500 \div 1500 \div 3000$

$= 1.111$

Answer $= $ **1.1 (tenth)** or **1.11 (hundredth)**

Option 2: Initial Reduction of Fractions

$$\frac{2000}{1500} \times \frac{2500}{3000}$$

$$\frac{\overset{2}{\cancel{2000}}}{\underset{3}{\cancel{1500}}} \times \frac{\overset{5}{\cancel{2500}}}{\underset{3}{\cancel{3000}}}$$

$$2 \times 5 \div 3 \div 3$$

$$= 1.111$$

Answer = **1.1 (tenth)** or **1.11 (hundredth)**

Problems 3.1

**Solve the equations. Express answers to the nearest tenth and hundredth.
A calculator may be used.**

1. $\dfrac{3}{8} \times \dfrac{6}{3}$ = _____ _____

2. $\dfrac{3}{4} \times \dfrac{10}{2}$ = _____ _____

3. $\dfrac{3}{5} \times \dfrac{1050}{40}$ = _____ _____

4. $\dfrac{10}{1} \times \dfrac{750}{40,000} \times \dfrac{1000}{1} \times \dfrac{1}{60}$ = _____ _____

5. $\dfrac{12}{1} \times \dfrac{500}{2700} \times \dfrac{2000}{1} \times \dfrac{1}{60}$ = _____ _____

6. $\dfrac{1500}{750} \times \dfrac{350}{600}$ = _____ _____

7. $\dfrac{1000}{2700} \times \dfrac{1300}{500} \times \dfrac{70}{50}$ = _____ _____

8. $\dfrac{15}{1} \times \dfrac{2500}{20,000} \times \dfrac{1000}{1} \times \dfrac{1}{60}$ = _____ _____

9. $\dfrac{8}{1} \times \dfrac{1000}{5000} \times \dfrac{100}{1} \times \dfrac{1}{60}$ = _____ _____

10. $\dfrac{750}{500} \times \dfrac{250}{300}$ = _____ _____

Answers **1.** 0.8; 0.75 **2.** 3.8; 3.75 **3.** 15.8; 15.75 **4.** 3.1; 3.13 **5.** 74.1; 74.07 **6.** 1.2; 1.17
7. 1.3; 1.35 **8.** 31.3; 31.25 **9.** 2.7; 2.67 **10.** 1.3; 1.25

DECIMAL FRACTION EQUATIONS

Decimal fraction equations raise an instant warning flag in calculations, because it is here that most dosage errors occur. As with whole-number equations, simplifying the numbers by eliminating decimal points and reducing the numbers is an optional first step. If you elect to do the entire calculation with a calculator, be sure to enter the decimal points carefully. Double-check all calculator entries and answers.

Particular care must be taken with calculator entry of decimal numbers to include the decimal point. Each entry and answer must be routinely double-checked.

EXAMPLE 1

Option 1: Calculator Use Throughout

$$\frac{0.3}{1.65} \times \frac{2.5}{1}$$

$0.3 \times 2.5 \div 165$ Multiply 0.3 by 2.5, then divide by 1.65

$= 0.454$

Answer $=$ **0.5 (tenth)** or **0.45 (hundredth)**

Option 2: Initial Elimination of Decimal Points and Reduction of Fractions

$$\frac{0.3}{1.65} \times \frac{2.5}{1}$$

$$\frac{30}{165} \times \frac{25}{10}$$ Move the decimal point two places in 0.3 and 1.65 (to become 30 and 165) and one place in 2.5 and 1 (to become 25 and 10)

$$\frac{\overset{3}{\cancel{30}}}{\underset{33}{\cancel{165}}} \times \frac{\overset{5}{\cancel{25}}}{\underset{1}{\cancel{10}}}$$ Divide 30 and 10 by 10, then divide 25 and 165 by 5

$$\frac{\overset{1}{\cancel{3}}}{\underset{11}{\cancel{33}}} \times \frac{5}{1}$$ Divide 3 and 33 by 3

$5 \div 11$ Divide the remaining numerator, 5, by the denominator, 11

$= 0.454$

Answer $=$ **0.5 (tenth)** or **0.45 (hundredth)**

EXAMPLE 2

Option 1: Calculator Use Throughout

$$\frac{0.3}{1.2} \times \frac{2.1}{0.15}$$

$0.3 \times 2.1 \div 1.2 \div 0.15$ Multiply 0.3 by 2.1, then divide by 1.2 and 0.15

$= 3.5$

Answer $=$ **3.5 (tenth)** or **3.5 (hundredth)**

Option 2: Initial Elimination of Decimal Points and Reduction of Fractions

$$\frac{0.3}{1.2} \times \frac{2.1}{0.15}$$

$$\frac{3}{12} \times \frac{210}{15}$$ Eliminate the decimal points by moving them one place in 0.3 and 1.2 (to become 3 and 12) and two places in 2.1 and 0.15 (to become 210 and 15)

$$\frac{\overset{1}{\cancel{3}}}{\underset{4}{\cancel{12}}} \times \frac{\overset{42}{\cancel{210}}}{\underset{3}{\cancel{15}}}$$ Divide 3 and 12 by 3, then divide 210 and 15 by 5

$$\frac{1}{\underset{2}{\cancel{4}}} \times \frac{\overset{21}{\cancel{42}}}{3}$$ Divide 42 and 4 by 2

$21 \div 2 \div 3$ Use a calculator to divide the numerator, 21, by 2 and then by 3

$= 3.5$

Answer = **3.5 (tenth)** or **3.5 (hundredth)**

EXAMPLE 3 **Option 1: Calculator Use Throughout**

$$\frac{0.15}{0.17} \times \frac{3.1}{2}$$

$0.15 \times 3.1 \div 0.17 \div 2$ Multiply 0.15 by 3.1, divide by 0.17, and then divide by 2

$= 1.367$

Answer = **1.4 (tenth)** or **1.37 (hundredth)**

Option 2: Initial Elimination of Decimal Points and Reduction of Fractions

$$\frac{0.15}{0.17} \times \frac{3.1}{2}$$

$$\frac{15}{17} \times \frac{31}{20}$$ Move the decimal point two places in 0.15 and 0.17 and one place in 3.1 and 2 (requires adding a zero to 2)

$$\frac{\overset{3}{\cancel{15}}}{17} \times \frac{31}{\underset{4}{\cancel{20}}}$$ Divide 15 and 20 by 5

$3 \times 31 \div 17 \div 4$ Complete this with a calculator

$= 1.367$

Answer = **1.4 (tenth)** or **1.37 (hundredth)**

EXAMPLE 4 **Option 1: Calculator Use Throughout**

$$\frac{2.5}{1.5} \times \frac{1.2}{1.1}$$

$2.5 \times 1.2 \div 1.5 \div 1.1$

$= 1.818$

Answer = **1.8 (tenth)** or **1.82 (hundredth)**

Option 2: Initial Elimination of Decimal Points and Reduction of Fractions

$$\frac{2.5}{1.5} \times \frac{1.2}{1.1}$$

$$\frac{25}{15} \times \frac{12}{11}$$

$$\frac{\overset{5}{\cancel{25}}}{\underset{3}{\cancel{15}}} \times \frac{12}{11}$$

$$\frac{5}{\underset{1}{\cancel{3}}} \times \frac{\overset{4}{\cancel{12}}}{11}$$

$$5 \times 4 \div 11$$

$$= 1.818$$

Answer = **1.8 (tenth)** or **1.82 (hundredth)**

Problems 3.2

Solve the equations. Express answers to the nearest tenth and hundredth. A calculator may be used.

1. $\dfrac{2.1}{1.15} \times \dfrac{0.9}{1.2}$ = _____ _____

2. $\dfrac{3.1}{2.7} \times \dfrac{2.2}{1.4}$ = _____ _____

3. $\dfrac{0.3}{1.2} \times \dfrac{3}{2.1}$ = _____ _____

4. $\dfrac{0.17}{0.3} \times \dfrac{2.5}{1.5}$ = _____ _____

5. $\dfrac{1.75}{0.95} \times \dfrac{1.5}{2}$ = _____ _____

6. $\dfrac{0.75}{1.15} \times \dfrac{3}{1.25}$ = _____ _____

7. $\dfrac{10.2}{1.5} \times \dfrac{2}{5.1}$ = _____ _____

8. $\dfrac{0.125}{0.25} \times \dfrac{2.5}{1.5}$ = _____ _____

9. $\dfrac{0.9}{0.3} \times \dfrac{1.2}{1.4}$ = _____ _____

10. $\dfrac{0.35}{1.7} \times \dfrac{2.5}{0.7}$ = _____ _____

Answers **1.** 1.4; 1.37 **2.** 1.8; 1.8 **3.** 0.4; 0.36 **4.** 0.9; 0.94 **5.** 1.4; 1.38 **6.** 1.6; 1.57 **7.** 2.7; 2.67 **8.** 0.8; 0.83 **9.** 2.6; 2.57 **10.** 0.7; 0.74

MULTIPLE-NUMBER EQUATIONS

The calculation steps just practiced are also used for multiple-number equations, which occur frequently in advanced clinical calculations. **Reduction of numbers may be of particular benefit here because calculations of this type sometimes have numbers that cancel and/or reduce dramatically.** Answers are expressed to the nearest whole number in the examples and problems that follow to replicate actual clinical calculations.

EXAMPLE 1   **Option 1: Calculator Use Throughout**

$$\frac{60}{1} \times \frac{1000}{4} \times \frac{1}{1000} \times \frac{6}{1}$$

$60 \times 1000 \times 6 \div 4 \div 1000$ Multiply 60 by 1000, then by 6;
divide by 4 and 1000

$= 90$

Answer $= $ **90**

Option 2: Initial Reduction of Fractions

$$\frac{60}{1} \times \frac{1000}{4} \times \frac{1}{1000} \times \frac{6}{1}$$

$$\frac{60}{1} \times \frac{\overset{1}{\cancel{1000}}}{\underset{2}{\cancel{4}}} \times \frac{1}{\underset{1}{\cancel{1000}}} \times \frac{\overset{3}{\cancel{6}}}{1}$$ Eliminate 1000 from a numerator and
denominator, then divide 6 and 4 by 2

$60 \times 3 \div 2$ Multiply 60 by 3, then divide by 2

$= 90$

Answer $= $ **90**   The answer is obtained by
cancellation alone

EXAMPLE 2   **Option 1: Calculator Use Throughout**

$$\frac{20}{1} \times \frac{75}{1} \times \frac{1}{60}$$

$20 \times 75 \div 60$ Multiply 20 by 75, then divide by 60

$= 25$

Answer $= $ **25**

Option 2: Initial Reduction of Fractions

$$\frac{20}{1} \times \frac{75}{1} \times \frac{1}{60}$$

$$\frac{\overset{1}{\cancel{20}}}{1} \times \frac{\overset{25}{\cancel{75}}}{1} \times \frac{1}{\underset{\underset{1}{3}}{\cancel{60}}}$$ Divide 20 and 60 by 20 to become 1 and 3, then
divide 75 and 3 by 3 to become 25 and 1

$= 25$

Answer $= $ **25**   The answer is obtained by cancellation alone

EXAMPLE 3   **Option 1: Calculator Use Throughout**

$$\frac{2}{0.5} \times \frac{1}{100} \times \frac{275}{1}$$

$2 \times 275 \div 0.5 \div 100$ Multiply 2 by 275, then divide by 0.5 and 100

$= 11$

Answer $= $ **11**

Option 2: Initial Reduction of Fractions

$$\frac{2}{0.5} \times \frac{1}{100} \times \frac{275}{1}$$

$$\frac{20}{5} \times \frac{1}{100} \times \frac{275}{1}$$

Eliminate the decimal point by moving it one place in 0.5 and one place in 2, which requires adding a zero to 2 (to become 5 and 20)

$$\frac{\overset{1}{\cancel{20}}}{\underset{1}{\cancel{5}}} \times \frac{1}{\underset{5}{\cancel{100}}} \times \frac{\overset{55}{\cancel{275}}}{1}$$

Divide 20 and 100 by 20, then divide 275 and 5 by 5

$$\frac{1}{\underset{1}{\cancel{5}}} \times \frac{\overset{11}{\cancel{55}}}{1}$$

Divide 5 and 55 by 5

$$= 11$$

Answer = **11**   The answer is obtained by cancellation alone

EXAMPLE 4   **Option 1: Calculator Use Throughout**

$$\frac{1}{60} \times \frac{1}{12} \times \frac{10}{1} \times \frac{750}{1}$$

$$10 \times 750 \div 60 \div 12$$

$$= 10.4$$

Answer = **10**

Option 2: Initial Reduction of Fractions

$$\frac{1}{60} \times \frac{1}{12} \times \frac{10}{1} \times \frac{750}{1}$$

$$\frac{1}{\underset{6}{\cancel{60}}} \times \frac{1}{\underset{6}{\cancel{12}}} \times \frac{\overset{1}{\cancel{10}}}{1} \times \frac{\overset{375}{\cancel{750}}}{1}$$

$$375 \div 6 \div 6$$

$$= 10.4$$

Answer = **10**

Problems 3.3

Solve the equations. Express answers to the nearest whole number.

1. $\dfrac{15}{1} \times \dfrac{350}{5} \times \dfrac{1}{60}$ = _____

2. $\dfrac{1}{32} \times \dfrac{60}{1} \times \dfrac{7.5}{3.1}$ = _____

3. $\dfrac{10}{1} \times \dfrac{2500}{24} \times \dfrac{1}{60}$ = _____

4. $\dfrac{1.7}{2.3} \times \dfrac{15.3}{12.1} \times \dfrac{6.2}{0.3}$ = _____

5. $\dfrac{20}{1} \times \dfrac{1200}{16} \times \dfrac{1}{60}$ = _____

6. $\dfrac{5}{1} \times \dfrac{320}{1.5} \times \dfrac{1}{60}$ = _____

7. $\dfrac{100}{1} \times \dfrac{1750}{200} \times \dfrac{1}{60}$ = _____

8. $\dfrac{60}{1} \times \dfrac{1150}{200} \times \dfrac{1}{100}$ = _____

9. $\dfrac{25}{4} \times \dfrac{1000}{8} \times \dfrac{1}{60} =$ _____

10. $\dfrac{18}{10} \times \dfrac{120}{7} \times \dfrac{9}{17} =$ _____

Answers   1. 18   **2.** 5   **3.** 17   **4.** 19   **5.** 25   **6.** 18   **7.** 15   **8.** 3   **9.** 13   **10.** 16

Summary

This concludes the chapter on solving common fraction equations. The important points to remember from this chapter are:

- Most clinical calculations consist of an equation containing one to five common fractions.

- In solving equations, all the numerators are multiplied, then divided by the denominators.

- Numbers in an equation may initially be reduced using common denominators/divisors to simplify final multiplication and division.

- Zeros may be eliminated from the same number of numerators and denominators without altering the value.

- Double-check all calculator entries and answers.

- Answers may be expressed as whole numbers, or to the nearest tenth or hundredth, depending on the calculation being done.

Summary Self-Test

Solve the equations. Express answers to the nearest tenth and hundredth. A calculator may be used.

1. $\dfrac{0.8}{0.65} \times \dfrac{1.2}{1} =$ _____ _____

2. $\dfrac{350}{1000} \times \dfrac{4.4}{1} =$ _____ _____

3. $\dfrac{0.35}{1.3} \times \dfrac{4.5}{1} =$ _____ _____

4. $\dfrac{0.4}{1.5} \times \dfrac{2.3}{1} =$ _____ _____

5. $\dfrac{1}{75} \times \dfrac{500}{1} =$ _____ _____

6. $\dfrac{0.15}{0.12} \times \dfrac{1.45}{1} =$ _____ _____

7. $\dfrac{100,000}{80,000} \times \dfrac{1.7}{1} =$ _____ _____

8. $\dfrac{1.45}{2.1} \times \dfrac{1.5}{1} =$ _____ _____

9. $\dfrac{1550}{500} \times \dfrac{0.5}{1} =$ _____ _____

10. $\dfrac{4}{0.375} \times \dfrac{0.25}{1} =$ _____ _____

11. $\dfrac{0.08}{0.1} \times \dfrac{2.1}{1} =$ _____ _____

12. $\dfrac{1.5}{1.25} \times \dfrac{1.45}{1}$ = _____ _____

13. $\dfrac{0.5}{0.15} \times \dfrac{0.35}{1}$ = _____ _____

14. $\dfrac{300,000}{200,000} \times \dfrac{1.7}{1}$ = _____ _____

15. $\dfrac{13.5}{10} \times \dfrac{1.8}{1}$ = _____ _____

16. $\dfrac{1,000,000}{800,000} \times \dfrac{1.4}{1}$ = _____ _____

17. $\dfrac{1.3}{0.2} \times \dfrac{0.25}{1}$ = _____ _____

18. $\dfrac{1.5}{0.1} \times \dfrac{0.25}{1}$ = _____ _____

19. $\dfrac{1.9}{3.5} \times \dfrac{3.2}{1.4}$ = _____ _____

20. $\dfrac{15,000}{7500} \times \dfrac{3.5}{1.2}$ = _____ _____

21. $\dfrac{4.7}{1.3} \times \dfrac{50}{20} \times \dfrac{4}{25} \times \dfrac{8.2}{2.1}$ = _____ _____

22. $\dfrac{40}{24} \times \dfrac{250}{5} \times \dfrac{0.375}{7.5}$ = _____ _____

23. $\dfrac{6.9}{21.6} \times \dfrac{250}{5} \times \dfrac{0.75}{2.1}$ = _____ _____

24. $\dfrac{1}{60} \times \dfrac{1}{25} \times \dfrac{10}{1} \times \dfrac{1000}{1}$ = _____ _____

25. $\dfrac{50.5}{22.75} \times \dfrac{4.7}{6.3} \times \dfrac{31.7}{10.2}$ = _____ _____

Solve the equations. Express answers to the nearest whole number. A calculator may be used.

26. $\dfrac{104}{95} \times \dfrac{20}{15} \times \dfrac{63}{1.6}$ = _____

27. $\dfrac{40,000}{10,000} \times \dfrac{30}{1} \times \dfrac{3.7}{12.5}$ = _____

28. $\dfrac{60}{1} \times \dfrac{500}{50} \times \dfrac{1}{1000} \times \dfrac{116}{1}$ = _____

29. $\dfrac{1.5}{0.6} \times \dfrac{10}{14} \times \dfrac{3.2}{5.3} \times \dfrac{100}{2}$ = _____

30. $\dfrac{60}{1} \times \dfrac{50}{250} \times \dfrac{1}{100} \times \dfrac{455}{1}$ = _____

31. $\dfrac{33.7}{15.9} \times \dfrac{19.2}{2.6} \times \dfrac{2.9}{3.85}$ = _____

32. $\dfrac{20}{4} \times \dfrac{100}{88} \times \dfrac{1200}{250} \times \dfrac{10}{30}$ = _____

33. $\dfrac{14}{7.9} \times \dfrac{88}{8}$ = _____

34. $\dfrac{10}{1} \times \dfrac{325}{1.5} \times \dfrac{1}{60}$ = _____

35. $\dfrac{60}{1} \times \dfrac{300}{400} \times \dfrac{1}{800} \times \dfrac{400}{1}$ = _____

36. $\dfrac{3.7}{1.3} \times \dfrac{12}{8} \times \dfrac{3.1}{7.4} \times \dfrac{5}{1}$ = _____

37. $\dfrac{20}{2} \times \dfrac{125}{25} \times \dfrac{2}{750} \times \dfrac{216}{1}$ = _____

38. $\dfrac{4}{3} \times \dfrac{45}{1} \times \dfrac{22.5}{37.8}$ = _____

39. $\dfrac{7.5}{12.3} \times \dfrac{55}{5} \times \dfrac{23.2}{1.2}$ = _____

40. $\dfrac{1000}{1} \times \dfrac{50}{250} \times \dfrac{20}{1} \times \dfrac{1}{60}$ = _____

41. $\dfrac{15}{1} \times \dfrac{1000}{4000} \times \dfrac{800}{1} \times \dfrac{1}{60}$ = _____

42. $\dfrac{15}{1} \times \dfrac{500}{3} \times \dfrac{1}{60}$ = _____

43. $\dfrac{25}{3} \times \dfrac{750}{8} \times \dfrac{0.1}{1}$ = _____

44. $\dfrac{40}{2} \times \dfrac{250}{50} \times \dfrac{1}{800} \times \dfrac{154}{1}$ = _____

45. $\dfrac{33}{4} \times \dfrac{75}{40} \times \dfrac{2}{150} \times \dfrac{432}{1}$ = _____

46. $\dfrac{22.5}{7} \times \dfrac{100}{5} \times \dfrac{1}{700} \times \dfrac{3}{80} \times \dfrac{3150}{1}$ = _____

47. $\dfrac{100}{250} \times \dfrac{50}{1} \times \dfrac{27.5}{1.375}$ = _____

48. $\dfrac{2.2}{0.25} \times \dfrac{3.6}{1} \times \dfrac{3.7}{7.1}$ = _____

49. $\dfrac{1.3}{0.21} \times \dfrac{0.3}{2} \times \dfrac{10.1}{0.75}$ = _____

50. $\dfrac{27.5}{10} \times \dfrac{40}{7} \times \dfrac{8.5}{1.9}$ = _____

Answers

1. 1.5; 1.48	**13.** 1.2; 1.17	**26.** 57	**39.** 130
2. 1.5; 1.54	**14.** 2.6; 2.55	**27.** 36	**40.** 67
3. 1.2; 1.21	**15.** 2.4; 2.43	**28.** 70	**41.** 50
4. 0.6; 0.61	**16.** 1.8; 1.75	**29.** 54	**42.** 42
5. 6.7; 6.67	**17.** 1.6; 1.63	**30.** 55	**43.** 78
6. 1.8; 1.81	**18.** 3.8; 3.75	**31.** 12	**44.** 19
7. 2.1; 2.13	**19.** 1.2; 1.24	**32.** 9	**45.** 89
8. 1; 1.04	**20.** 5.8; 5.83	**33.** 19	**46.** 11
9. 1.6; 1.55	**21.** 5.6; 5.65	**34.** 36	**47.** 400
10. 2.7; 2.67	**22.** 4.2; 4.17	**35.** 23	**48.** 17
11. 1.7; 1.68	**23.** 5.7; 5.7	**36.** 9	**49.** 13
12. 1.7; 1.74	**24.** 6.7; 6.67	**37.** 29	**50.** 70
	25. 5.1; 5.15	**38.** 36	

METRIC/ INTERNATIONAL (SI) SYSTEM

You are probably already familiar with the metric system, which is the major system of weights and measures used in medicine. The metric/international/SI (from the French Système International) system was invented in France in 1875, and takes its name from the meter, a length roughly equivalent to a yard, from which all other units of measure in the system are derived. The strength of the metric system lies in its simplicity, because all units of measure differ from each other in powers of ten (10). Conversions between units in the system are accomplished by simply moving a decimal point.

A major strength of the metric system is that all its units of measure differ from each other in powers of ten (10), and conversions between the units can be made by simply moving the decimal point.

This is also one of the metric system's greatest hazards. This is because a misplaced decimal point alters the value of a number by a multiple of at least 10. It is not necessary for you to know the entire metric system to administer medications safely, but you must understand its basic structure and become familiar with the units of measure you will be using in the clinical setting.

The greatest hazard of the metric system in drug dosages is that a misplaced decimal point will alter a dosage by a multiple of at least 10.

BASIC UNITS OF THE METRIC/SI SYSTEM

Three types of metric measures are in common clinical use: those for **length**, **volume** (or capacity), and **weight**. The basic units of these measures are:

> length — meter
> volume — liter
> weight — gram

Memorize the basic units if you do not already know them. In addition to the basic units, **there are both larger and smaller units of measure** for length, volume, and weight. Let's compare this concept with something familiar. The pound is a unit of weight that we use every day. A smaller unit of measure is the ounce; a larger, the ton. **However, all are units measuring weight.**

In the same way, there are smaller and larger units than the basic meter, liter, and gram. In the metric system, however, there is one very important advantage: **all other units, whether larger or smaller than the basic units, have the name of the basic unit incorporated in them.** So when you see a unit of metric measure, there is no doubt what it is measuring: **meter—length, liter—volume,** and **gram—weight.**

Problems 4.1

Identify the metric measures with their appropriate category of weight, length, or volume.

1. milligram _____

2. centimeter _____

3. milliliter _____

4. millimeter _____

5. kilogram _____

6. microgram _____

7. kilometer _____

8. kiloliter _____

Answers **1.** weight **2.** length **3.** volume **4.** length **5.** weight **6.** weight **7.** length **8.** volume

METRIC/SI PREFIXES

Prefixes are used in combination with the names of the basic units to identify larger and smaller units of measure. The same prefixes are used with all three measures. Therefore, there is a kilo**meter**, kilo**gram**, and a kilo**liter**.

Identical prefixes are used to identify units that are larger or smaller than the basic metric measures.

Prefixes also change the value of each of the basic units by the same amount. For example, the prefix "kilo" identifies a unit of measure that is larger than (or multiplies) the basic unit by 1000.

        1 kilometer = 1000 meters
        1 kilogram = 1000 grams
        1 kiloliter   = 1000 liters

Kilo is the only prefix you will be using in the clinical setting that identifies a measure **larger** than the basic unit. Kilograms are frequently used as a measure for body weight, especially for infants and children.

You will see only three measures **smaller** than the basic unit in common clinical use. The prefixes for these are:

        milli—as in milligram—for weight
        micro—as in microgram—for weight
        centi—as in centimeter—for length

Therefore, you will actually be working with only four prefixes: **kilo**, which identifies a larger unit of measure than the basic; and **milli**, **micro**, and **centi**, which identify smaller units than the basic.

METRIC/SI ABBREVIATIONS

In clinical use, units of metric measure are abbreviated.

 The basic units are abbreviated to their first initial and printed in small (lowercase) letters, with the exception of liter, which is capitalized (uppercase).

> meter is abbreviated **m**
>
> gram is abbreviated **g**
>
> liter is abbreviated **L**

 The abbreviations for the prefixes used in combination with the basic units are all printed using small letters.

> kilo is **k** (as in kilogram—kg)
>
> milli is **m** (as in milligram—mg)
>
> micro is **mc** (as in microgram—mcg)
>
> centi is **c** (as in centimeter—cm)

Micro has an additional abbreviation, the symbol μ, but its use has been discontinued in medication dosages. This became necessary because medication errors were made when handwritten μg was misread as mg, a dosage 1000 times the mcg dosage ordered.

 Micro is always abbreviated using the prefix mc rather than the symbol μ, which has an inherent safety risk.

In combination, liter remains capitalized. Therefore, milliliter is **mL** and kiloliter is **kL**.

Problems 4.2

Abbreviate the following metric units.

1. microgram   _____
2. liter   _____
3. kilogram   _____
4. milliliter   _____
5. centimeter   _____
6. milligram   _____
7. meter   _____
8. kiloliter   _____
9. millimeter   _____
10. gram   _____

Answers   **1.** mcg   **2.** L   **3.** kg   **4.** mL   **5.** cm   **6.** mg   **7.** m   **8.** kL   **9.** mm   **10.** g

METRIC/SI NOTATION RULES

To remember the rules of metric **notations**, in which **a unit of measure is expressed with a quantity**, it is helpful to memorize some prototypes (examples) that incorporate all the rules. For the metric system, the notations for one-half, one, and one and one-half milliliters incorporate all the official notation rules.

Prototype notations: **0.5 mL   1 mL   1.5 mL**

RULE 1   **The quantity is written in Arabic numerals: 1, 2, 3, 4, and so forth.**
Example: 0.5   1   1.5

RULE 2   **The numerals representing the quantity are placed in front of the abbreviations.**
Example: 0.5 mL   1 mL   1.5 mL   (**not** mL 0.5, mL 1, mL 1.5)

RULE 3   **A full space is used between the numeral and the abbreviation.**
Example: 0.5 mL   1 mL   1.5 mL   (**not** 0.5mL, 1mL, 1.5mL)

RULE 4   **Fractional parts of a unit are expressed as decimal fractions.**
Example: 0.5 mL   1.5 mL   (**not** ½ mL, 1½ mL)

RULE 5   **A zero is placed in front of the decimal when it is not preceded by a whole number to emphasize the decimal point.**
Example: 0.5 mL   (**not** .5 mL)

RULE 6   **Excess zeros following a decimal fraction are eliminated.**
Example: 0.5 mL   1 mL   1.5 mL   (**not** 0.50 mL, 1.0 mL, 1.50 mL)

Problems 4.3

Write the metric measures using official abbreviations and notation rules.

1. two grams   _____
2. five hundred milliliters   _____
3. five-tenths of a liter   _____
4. two-tenths of a milligram   _____
5. five-hundredths of a gram   _____
6. two and five-tenths kilograms   _____
7. one hundred micrograms   _____
8. two and three-tenths milliliters   _____
9. seven-tenths of a milliliter   _____
10. three-tenths of a milligram   _____
11. two and four-tenths liters   _____
12. seventeen and five-tenths kilograms   _____

13. nine-hundredths of a milligram _____

14. ten and two-tenths micrograms _____

15. four-hundredths of a gram _____

Answers 1. 2 g **2.** 500 mL **3.** 0.5 L **4.** 0.2 mg **5.** 0.05 g **6.** 2.5 kg **7.** 100 mcg **8.** 2.3 mL
9. 0.7 mL **10.** 0.3 mg **11.** 2.4 L **12.** 17.5 kg **13.** 0.09 mg **14.** 10.2 mcg **15.** 0.04 g

CONVERSION BETWEEN METRIC/SI UNITS

When you administer medications, you will be routinely **converting units of measure within the metric system;** for example, g to mg and mg to mcg. Learning the relative value of the units with which you will be working is the first prerequisite for accurate conversions.

There are only four metric **weights** commonly used in medicine. From **greater** to **lesser** value, these are:

kg = kilogram
g = gram
mg = milligram
mcg = microgram

Only two units of **volume** are frequently used. From **greater** to **lesser** value, these are:

L = liter
mL = milliliter

Each of these clinical metric measures differs from the next by 1000.

1 kg = 1000 g
1 g = 1000 mg
1 mg = 1000 mcg
1 L = 1000 mL

Once again, from greater to lesser value, the units are, for weight: kg—g—mg—mcg; for volume: L—mL. Each unit differs in value from the next by 1000, and **all conversions will be between touching units of measure;** for example, g to mg, mg to mcg, and L to mL.

Problems 4.4

Choose true (T) or false (F) for each conversion.

1. T F 1000 mL = 1000 L
2. T F 1000 mg = 1 g
3. T F 1000 g = 1 kg
4. T F 1000 mg = 1 mcg
5. T F 1000 mcg = 1 g
6. T F 1 kg = 1000 g
7. T F 1 mg = 1000 g
8. T F 1000 mcg = 1 mg
9. T F 1 g = 100 mcg
10. T F 1000 L = 1 kL

Answers 1. F **2.** T **3.** T **4.** F **5.** F **6.** T **7.** F **8.** T **9.** F **10.** T

Because the metric system is a decimal system, **conversions between the units are accomplished by moving the decimal point.** Also, because each unit of measure in clinical use differs from the next by 1000, if you know one conversion, you know them all.

How far do you move the decimal point? There is an unforgettable memory cue that can be used with **all** metric conversions. There are **three zeros in 1000.** The decimal point moves **three places**, the **same number of places as the zeros** in the conversion.

In metric conversions between touching units of clinical measures differing by 1000, the decimal point is moved three places, the same as the number of zeros in 1000.

This rule holds true for **all** decimal conversions in the metric system. If the difference in value was **10**, which has **one zero**, it would move **one place**. If the difference was **100**, which has **two zeros**, it would move **two places**. When the difference is **1000**, as in clinical conversions, which has **three zeros**, the decimal point moves **three places**.

Which way do you move the decimal point? If you are converting to a **smaller** unit of measure—for example, g to mg or L to mL—the **quantity must get larger.** The decimal point must move three places to the **right.**

EXAMPLE 1   0.5 g = _____ mg

You are converting to smaller units of measure, from **g to mg**, so the quantity will be **larger**. Move the decimal point **three places to the right.** To do this, you must **add two zeros** to the end of the quantity, and **eliminate the zero in front** of it. The larger 500 mg quantity indicates that you have moved the decimal point in the correct direction.

Answer   **0.5 g = .500. mg**   Move the decimal three places to the right

EXAMPLE 2   2.5 L = _____ mL

You are converting to smaller units of measure, so the quantity will be **larger.** Move the decimal point **three places to the right.** To do this, you must **add two zeros.** The larger 2500 mL quantity indicates that you have moved the decimal point in the correct direction.

Answer   **2.5 L = 2.500. mL**

Problems 4.5

Convert the metric measures.

1. 7 mg   = _____ mcg
2. 1.7 L   = _____ mL
3. 3.2 g   = _____ mg
4. 0.03 kg = _____ g
5. 0.4 mg   = _____ mcg

6. 1.5 mg   = _____ mcg
7. 0.7 g   = _____ mg
8. 0.3 L   = _____ mL
9. 7 kg   = _____ g
10. 0.01 mg = _____ mcg

Answers **1.** 7000 mcg **2.** 1700 mL **3.** 3200 mg **4.** 30 g **5.** 400 mcg **6.** 1500 mcg
7. 700 mg **8.** 300 mL **9.** 7000 g **10.** 10 mcg

In metric conversions from **smaller to larger units** of measurement, such as mL to L and mcg to mg, the quantity will be **smaller**. The decimal point is moved **three places to the left**.

EXAMPLE 1   200 mL = _____ L

You are converting to a larger unit of measure, **mL** to **L**, so the quantity will be **smaller**. Move the decimal point **three places to the left**.

.200. mL = .200 L

Eliminate the two unnecessary zeros at the end of the quantity (to make it .2), then add a zero in front of the decimal point to correctly write the dosage as 0.2 L.

Answer = **.200. mL = 0.2 L**

EXAMPLE 2   1500 mcg = _____ mg

You are converting to a larger unit of measure, so the quantity will be smaller. Move the decimal point **three places to the left. Place a decimal point in front of** the 5, and **eliminate the two zeros** after the 5.

Answer = **1.500. mcg = 1.5 mg**

EXAMPLE 3   300 mcg = _____ mg

You are converting to a larger unit of measure, **mcg** to **mg**, so the quantity will be **smaller**. Move the decimal point **three places to the left**.

.300. mcg = .300 mg

Two zeros will need to be eliminated from the end of this decimal fraction (to make it .3), and a zero must be placed in front of the decimal point to complete the decimal fraction.

Answer = **300 mcg = 0.3 mg**

Problems 4.6

Convert the metric measures.

1. 3500 mL = _____ L
2. 520 mg = _____ g
3. 1800 mcg = _____ mg
4. 750 mL = _____ L
5. 150 mg = _____ g

6. 250 mcg = _____ mg
7. 1200 mg = _____ g
8. 600 mL = _____ L
9. 100 mg = _____ g
10. 950 mcg = _____ mg

Answers   **1.** 3.5 L   **2.** 0.52 g   **3.** 1.8 mg   **4.** 0.75 L   **5.** 0.15 g   **6.** 0.25 mg   **7.** 1.2 g   **8.** 0.6 L
9. 0.1 g   **10.** 0.95 mg

COMMON ERRORS IN METRIC/SI DOSAGES

Most errors in the metric system occur because orders are not written using correct notation rules, or they are not transcribed correctly. **Errors usually involve decimal fractions.** Even though you have just finished learning metric notation rules, let's review the most common errors.

One error is the **failure to enter a zero in front of a decimal point**; for example, .2 mg instead of **0.**2 mg. Regardless of the presence of a zero in front of the decimal in a written order, one must be added when the order is transcribed to a medication administration record.

 Fractional dosages in the metric system are transcribed with a zero in front of the decimal point.

Another common error is to **include zeros where they should not be**; for example, 2.**0** mg instead of 2 mg or .**20** mg instead of 0.2 mg. Each error can be misread as 20 mg, a dosage greatly in excess of the intended dosage.

 Unnecessary zeros are eliminated when metric dosages are transcribed.

Errors are also more likely to occur in **calculations that include decimal fractions**. The presence of a decimal fraction in a calculation raises a warning flag to slow down and double-check all math. **Use your reasoning powers.** If a decimal is misplaced, the answer will be a minimum of 10 times too large or 10 times too small. **Question quantities that seem unreasonable.** A 1.5 mL IM injection dosage makes sense, but a 0.15 mL or 15 mL does not, and this is the type of error you might see.

 Question orders and calculations that seem unreasonably large or small.

Additional errors to be aware of are in **conversions within the metric system.** Errors in conversions can be eliminated by thinking **three.** All conversions between the g, mg, mcg, mL, and L measures are accomplished by moving the decimal point **three** places. Always and forever. There are not many things for which you can use the words "always" and "forever," but converting between these units of measure in the metric system is one of those rare instances.

 Conversions between g, mg, mcg, mL, and L units of measure in metric measures require moving the decimal point three places.

Be constantly mindful of these problem areas to become a safe clinical practitioner.

Summary

This concludes the refresher on the metric system. The important points to remember from this chapter are:

- The meter-m, liter-L, and gram-g are the basic units of metric measure.
- Only liter is capitalized, L.
- Larger and smaller units than the basics are identified by the use of prefixes.
- The prefixes are printed using small (lowercase) letters.
- The one larger unit you will be seeing is the kilo, whose prefix is k.
- The smaller units you will be seeing are milli—m, micro—mc, and centi—c.
- Each prefix changes the value of a basic unit by the same amount.
- Converting from one unit to another within the system is accomplished by moving a decimal point.
- When you convert from larger to smaller units of measurement, the quantity will increase.
- To convert from larger to smaller units, the decimal point is moved to the right.
- When you convert from smaller to larger units of measurement, the quantity will get smaller.
- To convert from smaller to larger units, the decimal point is moved to the left.
- Conversions between g to mg, mg to mcg, and mL to L all require moving the decimal point three places.
- Fractional dosages are transcribed with a zero in front of the decimal point.
- Unnecessary zeros are eliminated from dosages.

Summary Self-Test

List the basic units of measure of the metric system and the measure they are used for.

1. _____   _____

   _____   _____

   _____   _____

Identify the official metric/SI abbreviations.

2. a) L   e) mg

   b) g   f) kg

   c) kL   g) ml

   d) mgm   h) G

   _____

Use official metric abbreviations and notation rules to express these as numerals.

3. six-hundredths of a milligram   _____

4. three hundred and ten milliliters   _____

5. three-tenths of a kilogram   _____

6. four-tenths of a milliliter   _____

7. one and five-tenths grams   _____

8. one-hundredths of a gram   _____

9. four thousand milliliters   _____

10. one and two-tenths milligrams   _____

List the four commonly used clinical units of weight and the two of volume from greater to lesser value.

11. Weight   _____   _____   _____   _____

    Volume   _____   _____

Convert the metric measures.

12. 160 mg   = _____ g   27. 300 mg   = _____ g

13. 10 kg   = _____ g   28. 2.5 mg   = _____ mcg

14. 1500 mcg = _____ mg   29. 1 kL   = _____ L

15. 750 mg   = _____ g   30. 3 L   = _____ mL

16. 200 mL   = _____ L   31. 2 L   = _____ mL

17. 0.3 g   = _____ mg   32. 0.7 mg   = _____ mcg

18. 0.05 g   = _____ mg   33. 4 g   = _____ mg

19. 0.15 g   = _____ mg   34. 1000 mL   = _____ L

20. 1.2 L   = _____ mL   35. 2500 mL   = _____ L

21. 1800 mL   = _____ L   36. 1000 mg   = _____ g

22. 2 mg   = _____ mcg   37. 0.2 mg   = _____ mcg

23. 900 mcg   = _____ mg   38. 2000 g   = _____ kg

24. 2.1 L   = _____ mL   39. 1.4 g   = _____ mg

25. 475 mL   = _____ L   40. 2.5 L   = _____ mL

26. 0.9 L   = _____ mL

Answers			
	9. 4000 mL	**19.** 150 mg	**30.** 3000 mL
1. gram-weight;	**10.** 1.2 mg	**20.** 1200 mL	**31.** 2000 mL
liter-volume;	**11.** kg, g, mg, mcg,	**21.** 1.8 L	**32.** 700 mcg
meter-length	L, mL	**22.** 2000 mcg	**33.** 4000 mg
2. a, b, c, e, f	**12.** 0.16 g	**23.** 0.9 mg	**34.** 1 L
3. 0.06 mg	**13.** 10,000 g	**24.** 2100 mL	**35.** 2.5 L
4. 310 mL	**14.** 1.5 mg	**25.** 0.475 L	**36.** 1 g
5. 0.3 kg	**15.** 0.75 g	**26.** 900 mL	**37.** 200 mcg
6. 0.4 mL	**16.** 0.2 L	**27.** 0.3 g	**38.** 2 kg
7. 1.5 g	**17.** 300 mg	**28.** 2500 mcg	**39.** 1400 mg
8. 0.01 g	**18.** 50 mg	**29.** 1000 L	**40.** 2500 mL

5

UNIT, PERCENTAGE, MILLIEQUIVALENT, RATIO, HOUSEHOLD, AND APOTHECARY MEASURES

Objectives

The learner will recognize dosages:

1. measured in units.

2. measured as percentages.

3. using ratio strengths.

4. in milliequivalents.

5. in household measures.

6. in the apothecary system as obsolete.

Although metric measures predominate in medications, there are several other measures frequently used, particularly in parenteral (injectable) solutions, that are important for you to know. In addition, you must be familiar with several measures in the household system because you may occasionally see these.

INTERNATIONAL UNITS (units)

A number of drugs are measured in International Units. Insulin, penicillin, and heparin are commonly seen examples. Antibiotics, such as penicillin, have dosages in the hundredths of thousands and millions, and heparin has dosages in the thousandths. A unit **measures a drug in terms of its action**, not its physical weight. The word "units" is **not abbreviated; it is written in lower case using Arabic numerals in front of the measure**, with a space between; for example, 2000 units or 1,000,000 units. **Commas are not usually used in a quantity unless it has at least five numbers;** for example, 45,000 units.

Problems 5.1

Express the unit dosages in numerals.

1. two hundred and fifty thousand units   _____

2. ten units   _____

3. five thousand units   _____

4. forty-four units   _____

5. forty thousand units   _____

6. one million units   _____

7. one thousand units   _____

8. twenty-five hundred units   _____

9. thirty-four units   _____

10. one hundred units   _____

Answers 1. 250,000 units **2.** 10 units **3.** 5000 units **4.** 44 units **5.** 40,000 units
6. 1,000,000 units **7.** 1000 units **8.** 2500 units **9.** 34 units **10.** 100 units

PERCENTAGE (%) MEASURES

Percentage strengths are used extensively in intravenous solutions, and somewhat less commonly for a variety of other medications, including eye and topical (for external use) ointments. **Percentage (%) means parts per hundred. The greater the percentage strength, the stronger the solution or ointment**; for example, 3% is stronger than 1%. Fractional percentages are expressed as decimal fractions; for example, 0.45%. Notice that, unlike other written dosages, percentages are generally written with **no space between the quantity and percentage sign**.

In solutions, percent represents the number of grams of drug per 100 mL of solution.

EXAMPLE 1   100 mL of a 1% solution will contain 1 g of drug.

EXAMPLE 2   100 mL of a 2.5% solution will contain 2.5 g of drug.

EXAMPLE 3   100 mL of a 10% solution will contain 10 g of drug.

EXAMPLE 4   100 mL of a 0.9% solution will contain 0.9 g of drug.

These examples are included to point out that percentage solutions contain a significant amount of drug or other solute, and that reading percentage labels requires the same care as that used with other drug dosages.

MILLIEQUIVALENT (mEq) MEASURES

Milliequivalents (mEq) is **an expression of the number of grams of a drug contained in 1 mL of a normal solution**. This is a definition that is quite understandable to a pharmacist or chemist, but you need not memorize it. Milliequivalent dosages are also written using **Arabic numerals**, with a space between the **abbreviation that follows**, for example, 30 mEq. You will see milliequivalents used in a variety of oral and parenteral solutions, potassium chloride being a common intravenous example.

Problems 5.2

Express the milliequivalent dosages in numerals.

1. sixty milliequivalents   _____

2. fifteen milliequivalents   _____

3. forty milliequivalents   _____

4. one milliequivalent   _____

5. fifty milliequivalents   _____

6. eighty milliequivalents   _____

7. fifty-five milliequivalents   _____

8. seventy milliequivalents   _____

9. thirty milliequivalents   _____

10. twenty milliequivalents   _____

Answers **1.** 60 mEq **2.** 15 mEq **3.** 40 mEq **4.** 1 mEq **5.** 50 mEq **6.** 80 mEq **7.** 55 mEq
8. 70 mEq **9.** 30 mEq **10.** 20 mEq

RATIO MEASURES

Ratio strengths are used primarily in solutions. They represent **parts of drug per parts of solution**; for example, 1 : 1000 (one part drug to 1000 parts solution).

EXAMPLE 1 A 1 : 100 strength solution has 1 part drug in 100 parts solution.

EXAMPLE 2 A 1 : 5 solution contains 1 part drug in 5 parts solution.

EXAMPLE 3 A solution that is 1 part drug in 2 parts solution would be written 1 : 2

  The less solution a drug is dissolved in, the stronger the solution.

For example, a ratio strength of 1 : 10 (1 part drug to 10 parts solution) is much stronger than a 1 : 100 (1 part drug in 100 parts solution).

Ratio strengths are always expressed in their **simplest terms**. For example, 2 : 10 would be incorrect because it can be reduced to 1 : 5. Notice that ratio dosages are written separated by a colon, with a space between both numbers and the colon. Dosages using ratio strengths are not common, but you do need to know what they represent.

Problems 5.3

Express as ratios.

1. 1 part drug to 200 parts solution _____

2. 1 part drug to 4 parts solution   _____

3. 1 part drug to 7 parts solution   _____

Identify the strongest solution.

4. a) 1 : 20   b) 1 : 200   c) 1 : 2   _____

5. a) 1 : 50   b) 1 : 20   c) 1 : 100   _____

6. a) 1 : 1000   b) 1 : 5000   c) 1 : 2000   _____

Answers 1. 1 : 200 **2.** 1 : 4 **3.** 1 : 7 **4.** c **5.** b **6.** a

---

HOUSEHOLD AND APOTHECARY MEASURES

Household and apothecary measures are most often used in the home care setting, and their clinical use is becoming less frequent. The measures you may occasionally see include the **ounce, tablespoon, teaspoon, dram, and drop**. Abbreviations and/or names for all of these measures, except the drop, **still appear on many disposable medication cups**, and care must be taken not to confuse them with metric dosages. It is quite possible that these measures will be eliminated in the future because the health care industry has been moving rapidly to improve dosage labeling and medication abbreviation guidelines to reduce the possibility of errors.

The various abbreviations for household dosages and their metric equivalents are as follows:

Household Measure	Abbreviation	Metric Equivalent
ounce	oz	30 mL
tablespoon	T, TBS, tbs	15 mL
teaspoon	t, TSP, tsp	5 mL
dram	dr	4 mL
drop	gtt	1 mL

The volume of a drop depends on the size of the dropper being used.

A drop is so inaccurate a measure that medication droppers are now an integral part of small-volume liquid medication preparations. The use of drops is largely restricted to eye and ear drop use. One exception is in small-volume pediatric liquid medications, which are prepared with **integral medicine droppers that are calibrated by volume, or by actual dosage.**

APOTHECARY MEASURES

Apothecary measures are mentioned here only to point out that they are no longer used. However, in the event your instructor thinks that you must be familiar with these measures, please refer to Appendix 1 for a brief discussion of this system.

Summary

This concludes your introduction to the additional measures you will see used in dosages and in solutions. The important points to remember from this chapter are:

- International units measure a drug by its action rather than its weight.
- There is no abbreviation for units, which is written in full, units, in lower case letters.
- Percentage (%) strengths are frequently used in solutions and ointments.

▪ Percent represents grams of drug per 100 mL of solution.

▪ The greater the percentage strength, the stronger the solution.

▪ Milliequivalent is abbreviated mEq and is frequently used in solution measurements.

▪ Ratio strengths represent parts of drug per parts of solution.

▪ The smaller the volume of solution, the greater the ratio strength.

▪ T or tbs is the abbreviation for tablespoon (15 mL), and t or tsp for teaspoon (5 mL).

▪ The abbreviation gtt is used for drop, and oz for ounce.

▪ Apothecary measures are now obsolete and should not be used.

Summary Self-Test

Express the dosages using the official symbols/abbreviations.

1. three hundred thousand units _____

2. forty-five units _____

3. ten percent _____

4. two and a half percent _____

5. forty milliequivalents _____

6. a one in two thousand ratio _____

7. a one in ten ratio _____

8. one percent _____

9. one drop _____

10. two thousand units _____

11. five milliequivalents _____

12. nine-tenths percent _____

13. ten units _____

14. a one in two ratio _____

15. five percent _____

16. twenty milliequivalents _____

17. fourteen units _____

18. twenty percent _____

19. two million units _____

20. one hundred thousand units _____

Answers	**6.** 1 : 2000	**12.** 0.9%	**18.** 20%
1. 300,000 units	**7.** 1 : 10	**13.** 10 units	**19.** 2,000,000 units
2. 45 units	**8.** 1%	**14.** 1 : 2	**20.** 100,000 units
3. 10%	**9.** 1 gtt	**15.** 5%	
4. 2.5%	**10.** 2000 units	**16.** 20 mEq	
5. 40 mEq	**11.** 5 mEq	**17.** 14 units	

SECTION 3

Reading Medication Labels and Syringe Calibrations

ORAL MEDICATION LABELS AND DOSAGE CALCULATION

Objectives

The learner will:

1. identify scored tablets, unscored tablets, and capsules.

2. read drug labels to identify trade and generic names.

3. locate dosage strengths and calculate average dosages.

4. measure oral solutions using a medicine cup.

In this chapter, you will be introduced to labels of oral medications for both solid (tablet and capsule) and liquid (mL) medications. Medication label information includes trade and generic drug names, metric dosage strengths, manufacturer's name, and other details you need to be aware of, primarily so that you can quickly locate the correct dosage strength to calculate ordered dosages. You will then use actual drug labels to calculate a full range of oral medication dosages. **Average dosage calculations require only the information you have already learned on the metric system and in the Refresher Math Section on addition and subtraction**. They are routinely done mentally. Advanced calculations are needed primarily in clinical specialty areas, and they will be covered in later chapters.

> **Most oral dosages consist of one-half to three tablets or capsules, or one-half to double the mL volume of liquid medications, and are done mentally.**

We will begin with labels for solid drug preparations. These include tablets, scored tablets (which contain an indented marking to make breakage for partial dosages possible), enteric-coated tablets (which delay absorption until the drug reaches the small intestine), capsules (powdered or oily drugs in a gelatin cover), and sustained or controlled–release capsules (action spread over a prolonged period of time; for example, 12 hours). See illustrations in Figure 6-1.

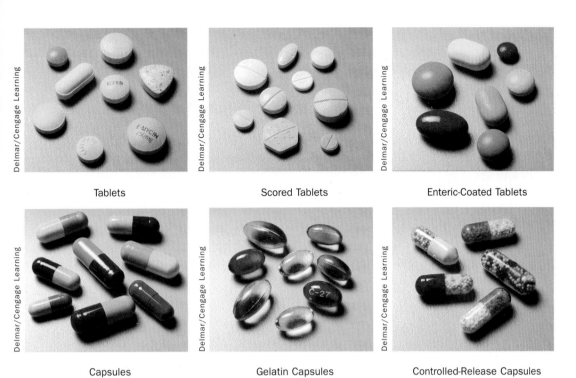

Tablets Scored Tablets Enteric-Coated Tablets

Capsules Gelatin Capsules Controlled-Release Capsules

Figure 6-1

TABLET AND CAPSULE LABELS

The most common type of label you will see in the clinical setting is the **unit dosage label**, in which each tablet or capsule is packaged separately. However, the dosage information on both unit and multiple dose labels is identical.

EXAMPLE 1

Look at the Synthroid® label in Figure 6-2. The first thing to notice is that this drug has two names. The first, **Synthroid**, is its **trade name**, which is identified by the ® registration symbol. Trade names are usually **capitalized** and **printed first** on the label. The name in smaller print, **levothyroxine sodium**, is the **generic** or

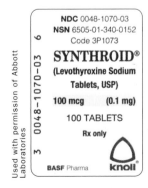

Figure 6-2

official name of the drug. Each drug has only **one** official name but may have **several trade names**, each for the exclusive use of the company that manufactures it. It is important to remember, however, that most labels do contain **both** names. Drugs may be ordered by either name depending on hospital policy or prescriber preference. You will frequently need to cross-check trade and generic names for accurate drug identification.

Next on the label is the **dosage strength**, 100 mcg or 0.1 mg. The prepared dosage is often representative of the **average dosage strength; the dosage given to the average patient at one time**. This label also identifies the **manufacturer** of this drug, Knoll Pharmaceuticals.

Notice that **100 TABLETS** is printed near the **bottom** of the label. This is the **total number** of tablets in the bottle. Be careful not to confuse the quantity of tablets or capsules with the dosage strength. **The dosage strength always has a unit of measure associated with it**; in this case, mcg and mg. Because label designs vary widely, this is an important point to remember.

EXAMPLE 2

The **Percocet®** label in Figure 6-3 is an example of a medication that contains not one but **two drugs**: 5 mg of the narcotic oxycodone and 325 mg of acetaminophen, an analgesic. The dosages in multiple drug products are routinely written in the same order as the drugs listed in the product. Oxycodone and acetaminophen are generic names, and Percocet is the manufacturer's trade name for this product. Medications that contain more than one drug are usually **ordered by trade name and number of tablets or capsules** to be given rather than by dosage.

The balance of the label information includes the total number of tablets near the bottom, 100; average dosage considerations; a bar code; and a space where the manufacturer would enter the drug lot number and expiration date. Expiration dates are carefully monitored by clinical pharmacies, but you must also make checking them a habit.

Tablets and capsules that contain more than one drug are usually ordered by trade name and number of tablets or capsules to be given, rather than by dosage.

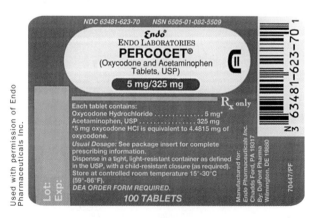

Figure 6-3

EXAMPLE 3

The small unit dosage label in Figure 6-4 bears only one name, **phenobarbital**, which is actually the **generic** name of the drug. Generic labeling is common with drugs that have been in use for generations. The official (generic) name was so well established that drug manufacturers did not try to promote their own trade names. Also notice that following the drug name are the initials **U.S.P.** This is the abbreviation for **U**nited **S**tates **P**harmacopeia, one of the two official national listings of drugs. The other is the **N**ational **F**ormulary, **NF.** You will see U.S.P. and NF on drug labels and must not confuse them with other initials that identify additional drugs or specific action of drugs in a preparation. Also notice that the label contains the dosage strength in both the metric, **15 mg**, and apothecaries, **1/4 gr**, measures. Finally, on the right of the label, printed sideways, is Exp 6-6-16, which identifies the last date when the drug should be used.

Next, refer to Figure 6-5. Notice that this label also contains the dosage strength of nitroglycerin in both the **0.3 mg metric** and the **1/200 gr (grains)** of the obsolete **apothecaries** system units of measure. As with phenobarbital, the inclusion of apothecaries dosages on this label relates to the age and historic use of this drug. Relabeling is already well under way by manufacturers to remove apothecaries dosages completely from their products.

 For safety in medication administration, focus on the drug name and its dosage strength.

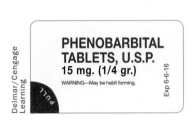

Figure 6-4

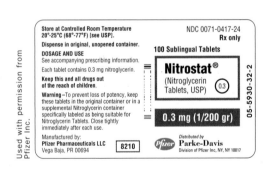

Figure 6-5

Problems 6.1

Refer to the label in Figure 6-5 and answer the questions about this drug.

1. What is the generic name? _____
2. What is the trade name? _____
3. What is the dosage strength in metric units? _____
4. What is the dosage strength in the obsolete apothecary measure? _____
5. If nitroglycerine 0.3 mg is ordered, how many tablets will be required? _____
6. Read the information above the Nitrostat name. What kind of tablets are these? _____

7. How must the drug be administered? _____

8. Who is the manufacturer of this drug? _____

9. How many tablets will be needed to give a 0.6 mg dosage of nitroglycerin? _____

Answers **1.** nitroglycerin **2.** Nitrostat® **3.** 0.3 mg **4.** 1/200 gr **5.** 1 tab **6.** sublingual **7.** under the tongue **8.** Parke Davis, a division of Pfizer Pharmaceuticals LLC **9.** 2 tab

---

Problems 6.2

Refer to the label in Figure 6-6 and answer the questions about this drug.

1. What is the generic name? _____

2. What is the trade name? _____

3. What is the dosage strength? _____

4. What company manufactured this drug? _____

5. How many tablets are in this container? _____

6. If Prinivil 5 mg is ordered, how many tablets will you give? _____

7. If lisinopril 10 mg is ordered, how many tablets will you give? _____

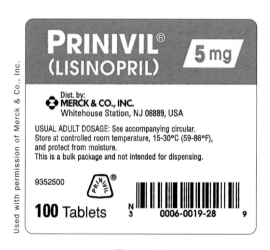

PRINIVIL® **5 mg**
(LISINOPRIL)

Dist. by:
✛ **MERCK & CO., INC.**
Whitehouse Station, NJ 08889, USA

USUAL ADULT DOSAGE: See accompanying circular.
Store at controlled room temperature, 15-30°C (59-86°F),
and protect from moisture.
This is a bulk package and not intended for dispensing.

9352500

100 Tablets   N 3   0006-0019-28   9

Used with permission of Merck & Co., Inc.

Figure 6-6

Answers **1.** lisinopril **2.** Prinivil® **3.** 5 mg **4.** Merck & Co., Inc. **5.** 100 tablets **6.** 1 tab **7.** 2 tab

---

Refer to the Sinemet® label in Figure 6-7. Sinemet is another example of a combined drug tablet. The **generic** names of the drugs it contains are **carbidopa** and **levodopa**. These are listed on the label in several places: directly under the trade name and with the **amount** of each drug in the fine print near the bottom of the label. Also, notice the box to the right of the trade name, which contains the numbers 25-100. This again is the amount of carbidopa—25 mg—and levodopa—100 mg. Contrast this label with the Sinemet labels in Figures 6-8 and 6-9.

In Figure 6-8, the dosage strengths are different. A blue box to the right of the Sinemet trade name identifies the strengths of carbidopa and levodopa as **10 mg** and **100 mg**, respectively, which are actually lower dosages. And, finally, Figure 6-9 is a label for Sinemet® **CR**, a **c**ontrolled-**r**elease or sustained-release tablet, with yet another dosage strength of 50-200: **carbidopa 50 mg** and **levodopa 200 mg**. Unlike the previous combined drug tablet discussed, an order for Sinemet **must** include the dosage because it is available in several strengths.

Extra numbers after a drug name may be used to identify the dosage strengths of more than one drug in a preparation, and extra initials may be used to identify a special drug action.

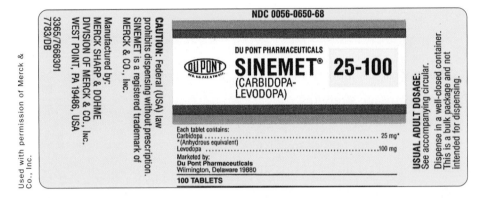

Figure 6-7

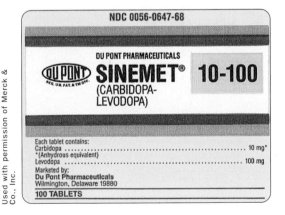

Figure 6-8

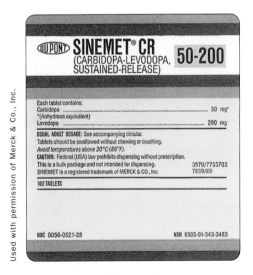

Figure 6-9

TABLET/CAPSULE DOSAGE CALCULATION

When the time comes for you to administer medications, you will have to read a **M**edication **A**dministration **R**ecord, abbreviated MAR, to prepare the dosage. This will tell you the name and amount of drug to be given, but it will not tell you how many tablets or capsules contain this dosage. This you must calculate yourself. However, remember that most tablets/capsules are prepared in average dosage strengths, and most orders will involve giving one-half to three tablets (or one to three capsules, since capsules cannot be broken in half). **Learn to question orders for more than three tablets or capsules.** Although some drugs require multiple tablets, most do not. Some clinical pharmacies do carry a limited quantity of a particular medication as a cost-saving factor, so if a drug came in 25 mg, 50 mg, 100 mg, and 200 mg dosages and that facility's pharmacy only carried 25 mg tablets, an order for 200 mg would translate into 8 tablets, which would seem unreasonable. In the 100 or 200 mg supply, the order results in 1 or 2 tablets, which is reasonable. Always question an order of more than 3 tablets, and double-check your calculations.

 An unusual number of tablets or capsules could be a warning of an error in prescribing, transcribing, or calculation.

Let's now look at some sample orders and do some actual dosage calculations. **Assume that tablets are scored and can be broken in half.**

Problems 6.3

Refer to the Inderal®LA label in Figure 6-10 to answer these questions.

1. What is the dosage strength?   _____
2. If you have an order for 120 mg, give   _____
3. If you have an order for 60 mg, give   _____
4. What is the generic name of this drug?   _____
5. What is the total number of capsules in this package?   _____

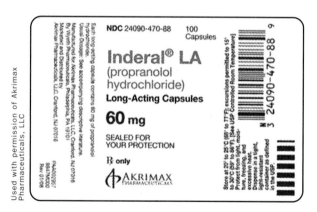

Figure 6-10

Answers   1. 60 mg   **2.** 2 cap   **3.** 1 cap   **4.** propranolol hydrochloride   **5.** 100 capsules

Problems 6.4

Refer to the Aricept® label in Figure 6-11 to answer these questions.

1. What is the dosage strength?   _____
2. If 10 mg is ordered, give   _____
3. If 2.5 mg is ordered, give   _____
4. If 5 mg is ordered, give   _____
5. What is the generic name of this drug?   _____
6. What is the total number of tablets in this package?   _____

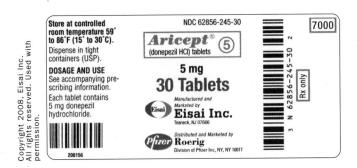

Figure 6-11

It is not uncommon to have a drug **ordered** in one unit of metric measure—**for example, mg**—and discover that it is **labeled** in another measure—**for example, g**. It will then be necessary to **convert the metric units to calculate the dosage**. Conversions will always be between touching units of measure: g and mg or mg and mcg. **Converting involves moving the decimal point three places**.

EXAMPLE 1

Refer to the Halcion® label in Figure 6-12. A dosage of 250 mcg has been ordered. The label reads 0.25 mg. Convert the mg to mcg by moving the decimal point three places to the right, and you can mentally verify that these dosages are identical. Give 1 tablet.

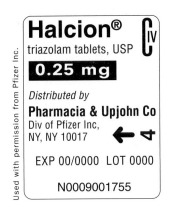

Figure 6-12

EXAMPLE 2

Refer to the Klonopin® label in Figure 6-13. A dosage of 1000 mcg is ordered. The label reads 0.5 mg, so you must give 2 tablets (1 tab = 500 mcg, so 1000 mcg requires 2 tab). The decimal moves three places to the right in this conversion from mg to mcg.

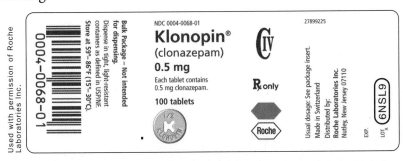

Figure 6-13

Problems 6.5

Locate the appropriate labels for the following dosages, and indicate how many tablets or capsules are needed to give them. Assume all tablets are scored and can be broken in half. Labels may be used in more than one problem.

1. verapamil HCl 0.12 g   _____ cap
2. Terbutaline® 10 mg   _____ tab
3. Ritalin® HCl 7.5 mg   _____ tab
4. methyphenidate HCl 2500 mcg   _____ tab

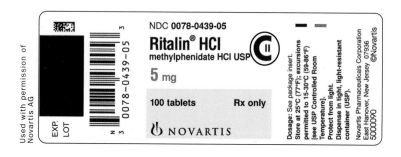

Used with permission of Novartis AG

NDC 0078-0439-05

Ritalin® HCl
methylphenidate HCl USP   C II

5 mg

100 tablets   Rx only

Ⓤ NOVARTIS

0078-0439-05

EXP.
LOT

Dosage: See package insert.
Store at 25°C (77°F); excursions permitted to 15-30°C (59-86°F) [see USP Controlled Room Temperature].
Protect from light.
Dispense in tight, light-resistant container (USP).

Novartis Pharmaceuticals Corporation
East Hanover, New Jersey 07936
5000090   ©Novartis

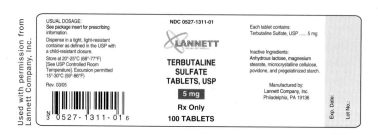

Used with permission from Lannett Company, Inc.

USUAL DOSAGE:
See package insert for prescribing information.
Dispense in a tight, light-resistant container as defined in the USP with a child-resistant closure.
Store at 20°-25°C (68°-77°F) [See USP Controlled Room Temperature]. Excursion permitted 15°-30°C (59°-86°F)
Rev. 03/05

NDC 0527-1311-01

✕ LANNETT

**TERBUTALINE
SULFATE
TABLETS, USP**

5 mg

Rx Only
100 TABLETS

3 0527-1311-01 6

Each tablet contains:
Terbutaline Sulfate, USP ...... 5 mg

Inactive Ingredients:
Anhydrous lactose, magnesium stearate, microcrystalline cellulose, povidone, and pregelatinized starch.

Manufactured by:
Lannett Company, Inc.
Philadelphia, PA 19136

Exp. Date:

Lot No.:

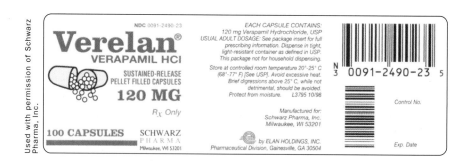

Used with permission of Schwarz Pharma, Inc.

NDC 0091-2490-23

Verelan®
VERAPAMIL HCl

SUSTAINED-RELEASE
PELLET FILLED CAPSULES

120 MG

Rₓ Only

100 CAPSULES   SCHWARZ
PHARMA
Milwaukee, WI 53201

EACH CAPSULE CONTAINS:
120 mg Verapamil Hydrochloride, USP
USUAL ADULT DOSAGE: See package insert for full prescribing information. Dispense in tight, light-resistant container as defined in USP. This package not for household dispensing.
Store at controlled room temperature 20°-25° C (68°-77° F) [See USP]. Avoid excessive heat. Brief digressions above 25° C, while not detrimental, should be avoided.
Protect from moisture.   L3795 10/98

Manufactured for:
Schwarz Pharma, Inc.
Milwaukee, WI 53201

℮ by ELAN HOLDINGS, INC.
Pharmaceutical Division, Gainesville, GA 30504

3 0091-2490-23 5

Control No.

Exp. Date

Problems 6.6

Locate the appropriate labels for the following drug orders, and indicate the number of tablets/capsules that will be required to administer the dosages ordered. Assume that all tablets are scored and can be broken in half. Notice that both generic and trade names are used for the orders and that a label may be used in more than one problem.

1. isosorbide dinitrate 80 mg   _____ cap

2. sulfasalazine 0.5 g   _____ tab

3. Azulfidine® 1 g   _____ tab

4. terbutaline sulfate 2500 mcg   _____ tab

5. chlordiazepoxide HCl 50 mg   _____ cap

6. Librium® 25 mg   _____ cap

7. Dilatrate®–SR 80 mg   _____ cap

8. Synthroid® 0.2 mg   _____ tab

9. levothyroxine Na 0.2 mg   _____ tab

10. terbutaline sulfate 3.75 mg   _____ tab

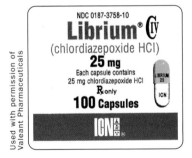

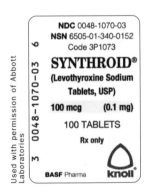

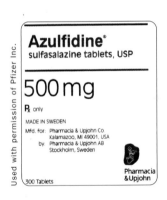

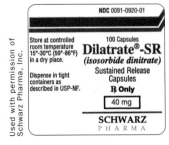

Answers **1.** 2 cap **2.** 1 tab **3.** 2 tab **4.** 1 tab **5.** 2 cap **6.** 1 cap **7.** 2 cap **8.** 2 tab **9.** 2 tab **10.** 1½ tab

ORAL SOLUTION LABELS

In liquid drug preparations, the dosage is contained in a certain mL **volume of solution**. Let's review dosages in some solid and liquid drug preparations to illustrate the difference.

EXAMPLE 1   **Solid** 250 mg in **1 tablet**   **Liquid:** 250 mg in **5 mL**

EXAMPLE 2   **Solid:** 100 mg in **1 capsule**   **Liquid:** 100 mg in **10 mL**

EXAMPLE 3

Refer to the Lomotil® label in Figure 6-14. The information it contains will be familiar. **Lomotil** is the **trade** name and **diphenoxylate** is the **generic** or official name. The dosage strength is **2.5 mg per 5 mL**. As with solid drugs, the medication administration record, MAR, will tell you the **dosage of the drug** to be administered, but it **will not specify the volume that contains this dosage**.

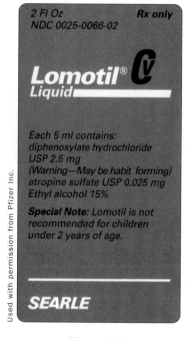

Figure 6-14

Used with permission from Pfizer Inc.

Problems 6.7

Refer to the Lomotil® label in Figure 6-14 to calculate these dosages.

1. The order is for diphenoxylate 2.5 mg. Give _____

2. The order is for Lomotil 5 mg. Give _____

Problems 6.8

Refer to the Penicillin® V label in Figure 6-15 to calculate these dosages.

1. The order is for Penicillin V 400,000 units.   _____

2. Penicillin V 125 mg has been ordered.   _____

3. Penicillin V 375 mg has been ordered.   _____

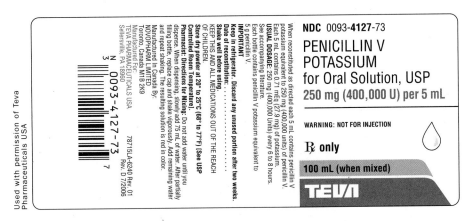

Figure 6-15

Problems 6.9

Refer to the solution labels in Figures 6-16 and 6-17 to calculate these dosages.

1. Prozac® soln. 10 mg   _____

2. cefaclor susp. 187 mg   _____

3. cefaclor susp. 374 mg   _____

4. fluoxetine HCl soln. 30 mg   _____

5. Prozac® soln. 40 mg _____

6. fluoxetine HCl soln. 20 mg _____

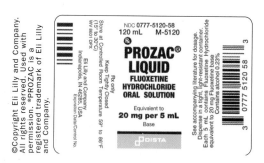

Figure 6-16

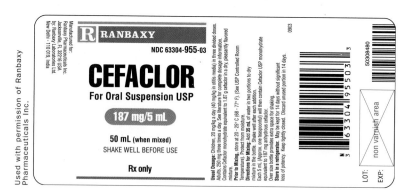

Figure 6-17

Answers   **1.** 2.5 mL   **2.** 5 mL   **3.** 10 mL   **4.** 7.5 mL   **5.** 10 mL   **6.** 5 mL

MEASUREMENT OF ORAL SOLUTIONS

Oral solutions are most commonly measured using a disposable **calibrated medication cup**. Take a close look at the schematic drawing of the medication cup calibrations in Figure 6-18. Many disposable medication cups, like this one, still contain the TSP (teaspoon), TBS (tablespoon), and OZ (ounce) calibrations of the household system and the obsolete DR (for dram) of the apothecaries system. Some also contain the increasingly disused cc (cubic centimeter) calibration, which is identical to a mL. Oral solutions are **most safely poured at eye level**. Because of the number of units of measure on these cups, **always read calibrations very carefully**.

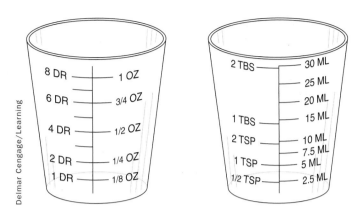

Figure 6-18

Small-volume solution dosages can also be measured using specially calibrated **oral syringes** such as those illustrated in Figures 6-19 and 6-20. Oral syringes have safety features built into their design to prevent their being mistaken for hypodermic syringes. One of these features is **color**, as illustrated in Figure 6-19. Hypodermic syringes are not colored, although their packaging and needle covers are colored to aid in identification. A second feature is the syringe tip, which is a **different size and shape** and is often **off center (termed eccentric)**. Figure 6-20 illustrates an eccentric oral syringe tip. Hypodermic syringes **without a needle** can also be used to measure and administer oral dosages.

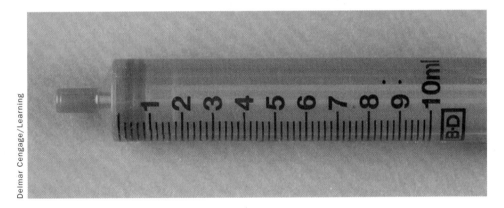

Figure 6-19

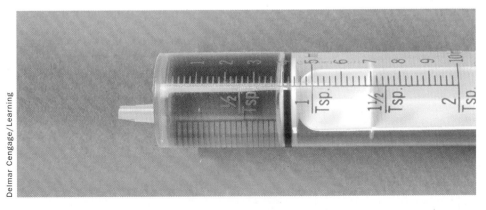

Figure 6-20

The main concern with correct syringe identification is that **oral syringes, which are not sterile**, should not be confused and used for **hypodermic medications, which are sterile.** This mistake **has** been made in spite of the fact that hypodermic needles do not fit correctly on oral syringes. The precaution, therefore, does need to be stressed.

Oral solutions may also be ordered as drops (gtt), and when this is the case, the dropper is attached to the bottle stopper. Medicine droppers are often calibrated in mL or by actual dosage, such as 125 mg, and so forth. (Refer to Chapter 20 for more information on droppers.)

Summary

This concludes the chapter on reading oral medication labels. The important points to remember from this chapter are:

- Most labels contain both generic and trade names.

- Dosages are clearly printed on the label, including preparations containing multiple drugs.

- Combined dosage tablets and capsules may be ordered by trade name and number of tablets/capsules to be given and may include dosages.

- The letters U.S.P. (United States Pharmacopeia) and NF (National Formulary) on drug labels identify their official generic listings.

- Additional letters that follow a drug name are used to identify additional drugs in the preparation or a special action of the drug.

- Most dosages of tablets or capsules consist of one-half to three tablets (1–3 capsules, which cannot be broken in half). An unusual number of tablets or capsules may indicate an error.

- Check expiration dates on labels before use.

- For accurate measurement, solutions are poured at eye level when a medicine cup is used.

- Liquid oral medications may be measured and administered using an oral medication syringe or a hypodermic syringe without a needle.

- Care must be taken not to use oral syringes for hypodermic medication preparation because these are not sterile.

Summary Self-Test

Locate the appropriate label for each of the following drug orders, and indicate the number of tablets, capsules, or mL that will be required to administer them. Assume that all tablets are scored and can be broken in half. Labels may be used more than once in each problem set.

PART I

1. Glucotrol® 15 mg   _____

2. dexamethasone 4 mg   _____

3. Dilatrate®-SR 80 mg   _____

4. morphine sulfate 20 mg   _____

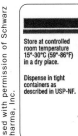

NDC 0091-0920-01

Store at controlled
room temperature
15°-30°C (59°-86°F)
in a dry place.

Dispense in tight
containers as
described in USP-NF.

100 Capsules

Dilatrate®-SR
(isosorbide dinitrate)
Sustained Release
Capsules
℞ Only

40 mg

SCHWARZ
P H A R M A

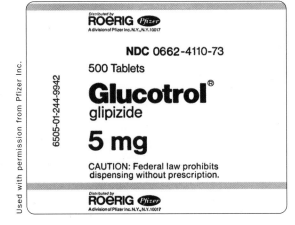

Distributed by
ROERIG *Pfizer*
A division of Pfizer Inc. N.Y., N.Y.10017

NDC 0662-4110-73

500 Tablets

Glucotrol®
glipizide

5 mg

CAUTION: Federal law prohibits
dispensing without prescription.

Distributed by
ROERIG *Pfizer*
A division of Pfizer Inc. N.Y., N.Y.10017

6505-01-244-9942

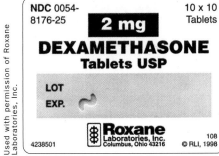

NDC 0054-
8176-25

2 mg

10 x 10
Tablets

DEXAMETHASONE
Tablets USP

LOT

EXP.

Roxane
Laboratories, Inc.
Columbus, Ohio 43216

4238501

108
© RLI, 1998

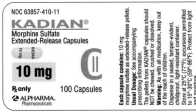

NDC 63857-410-11

KADIAN®
Morphine Sulfate
Extended-Release Capsules

10 mg

℞ only   100 Capsules

ALPHARMA.
Pharmaceuticals

Each capsule contains: 10 mg
morphine sulfate as extended-release pellets.
Usual Dosage: See accompanying
prescribing information.
The pellets from KADIAN® capsules should
NOT be chewed, crushed or dissolved.
Warning: As with all medication, keep out
of the reach of children.
Dispense in a sealed, tamper-evident,
childproof, light-resistant container.
Store at 25°C (77°F); excursions permitted
to 15°-30°C (59°-86°F). Protect from light
and moisture.

Manufactured for:
Alpharma Pharmaceuticals LLC
One New England Avenue
Piscataway, NJ 08854
by: Actavis Elizabeth LLC, 200 Elmora Avenue
Elizabeth, NJ 07207 USA   Rev. 04/07

Lot No.:

63857-410-11

PART II

5. piroxicam 20 mg   _____

6. cefaclor susp. 250 mg   _____

7. Lortab® 5/500 2 tab   _____

8. Halcion® 250 mcg   _____

9. alprazolam 750 mcg   _____

10. gabapentin 0.2 g   _____

11. Biaxin® 1 g   _____

12. Xanax® 500 mcg   _____

13. clarithromycin 0.5 g   _____

14. triazolam 500 mcg   _____

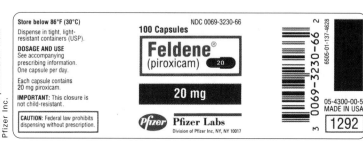

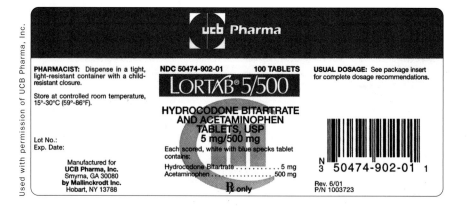

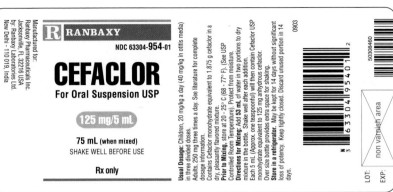

Manufactured for:
Ranbaxy Pharmaceuticals Inc.
Jacksonville, FL 32216 USA
by: Ranbaxy Laboratories Ltd.
New Delhi - 110 019, India

R̶ RANBAXY
NDC 63304-**954**-01

CEFACLOR
For Oral Suspension USP

125 mg/5 mL

75 mL (when mixed)
SHAKE WELL BEFORE USE

Rx only

Usual Dosage: Children, 20 mg/kg a day (40 mg/kg in otitis media) in three divided doses.
Adults, 250 mg three times a day. See literature for complete dosage information.
Contains Cefaclor monohydrate equivalent to 1.875 g cefaclor in a dry, pleasantly flavored mixture.
Prior to Mixing, store at 20 - 25° C (68 - 77° F). (See USP Controlled Room Temperature). Protect from moisture.
Directions for Mixing: Add 53 mL of water in two portions to dry mixture in the bottle. Shake well after each addition.
Each 5 mL (Approx. one teaspoonful) will then contain Cefaclor USP monohydrate equivalent to 125 mg anhydrous cefaclor.
Over size bottle provides extra space for shaking.
Store in a refrigerator. May be kept for 14 days without significant loss of potency. Keep tightly closed. Discard unused portion in 14 days.

0903

50308460

N 3 6 3 3 0 4 9 5 4 0 1 2

LOT:
EXP:

non varnish area

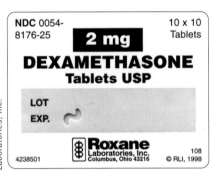

NDC 0054-
8176-25

2 mg

10 x 10
Tablets

DEXAMETHASONE
Tablets USP

LOT

EXP.

⊕ Roxane
Laboratories, Inc.
Columbus, Ohio 43216
© RLI, 1998

4238501

108

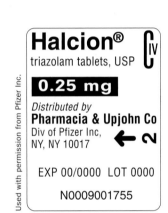

Halcion® C̶ IV
triazolam tablets, USP

0.25 mg

Distributed by
Pharmacia & Upjohn Co
Div of Pfizer Inc,
NY, NY 10017   ← 2

EXP 00/0000 LOT 0000

N0009001755

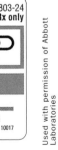 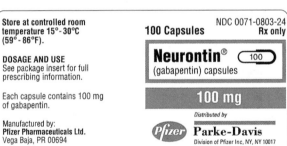

Store at controlled room
temperature 15°- 30°C
(59°- 86°F).

DOSAGE AND USE
See package insert for full
prescribing information.

Each capsule contains 100 mg
of gabapentin.

Manufactured by:
Pfizer Pharmaceuticals Ltd.
Vega Baja, PR 00694

100 Capsules

NDC 0071-0803-24
Rx only

Neurontin® (100)
(gabapentin) capsules

100 mg

Distributed by
Pfizer Parke-Davis
Division of Pfizer Inc, NY, NY 10017

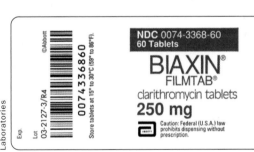

©Abbott

0074336860

Store tablets at 15° to 30°C (59° to 86°F).

Exp.

Lot
03-2127-3/R4

NDC 0074-3368-60
60 Tablets

BIAXIN®
FILMTAB®
clarithromycin tablets

250 mg

A̶B̶B̶ Caution: Federal (U.S.A.) law
prohibits dispensing without
prescription.

6505-01-354-8582
Do not accept if break-away
ring on cap is broken or missing.
Dispense in a USP tight, light-
resistant container.
Each tablet contains:
250 mg clarithromycin.
Each yellow tablet bears the 包
and Abbo-Code KT for product
identification.
Usual Adult Dose: One or two
tablets every twelve hours. See
enclosure for full prescribing
information.
Filmtab – Film-sealed tablets,
Abbott.
Abbott Laboratories
North Chicago, IL 60064, U.S.A.

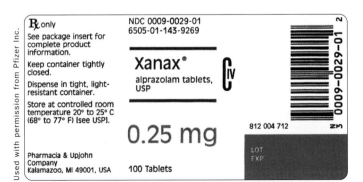

R̶ only
See package insert for
complete product
information.

Keep container tightly
closed.

Dispense in tight, light-
resistant container.

Store at controlled room
temperature 20° to 25° C
(68° to 77° F) (see USP).

Pharmacia & Upjohn
Company
Kalamazoo, MI 49001, USA

NDC 0009-0029-01
6505-01-143-9269

Xanax®
alprazolam tablets,
USP   C̶ IV

0.25 mg

812 004 712

100 Tablets

0009-0029-01

N 3   2

LOT
EXP

PART III

15. acetaminophen 650 mg   _____

16. Aldactone® 75 mg   _____

17. meclizine HCl 50 mg   _____

18. Kadian® 20 mg   _____

19. ciprofloxacin HCl 0.375 g   _____

20. metoprolol tartrate 0.15 g   _____

21. nifedipine 10 mg   _____

22. piroxicam 20 mg   _____

23. Feldene® 40 mg   _____

24. Lomotil® 2.5 mg   _____

25. Librium® 75 mg   _____

26. codeine 45 mg   _____

27. Aldactone® 50 mg   _____

28. Synthroid® 225 mcg   _____

29. nitroglycerin 600 mcg   _____

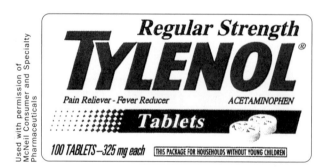

Used with permission of McNeil Consumer and Specialty Pharmaceuticals

Regular Strength
TYLENOL®
Pain Reliever - Fever Reducer   ACETAMINOPHEN
Tablets
100 TABLETS—325 mg each   THIS PACKAGE FOR HOUSEHOLDS WITHOUT YOUNG CHILDREN

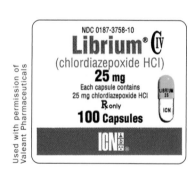

Used with permission of Valeant Pharmaceuticals

NDC 0187-3758-10
Librium® C IV
(chlordiazepoxide HCl)
25 mg
Each capsule contains
25 mg chlordiazepoxide HCl
R only
100 Capsules
ICN

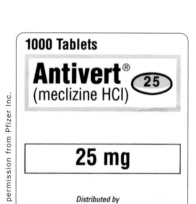

Used with permission from Pfizer Inc.

1000 Tablets
Antivert® 25
(meclizine HCl)
25 mg
Distributed by
Pfizer Roerig
Division of Pfizer Inc, NY, NY 10017

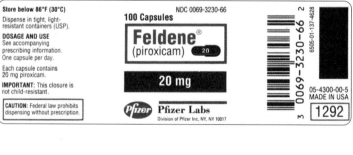

Used with permission from Pfizer Inc.

Store below 86°F (30°C)
Dispense in tight, light-resistant containers (USP).
DOSAGE AND USE
See accompanying prescribing information. One capsule per day.
Each capsule contains 20 mg piroxicam.
IMPORTANT: This closure is not child-resistant.
CAUTION: Federal law prohibits dispensing without prescription.

NDC 0069-3230-66
100 Capsules
Feldene®
(piroxicam) 20
20 mg
Pfizer Pfizer Labs
Division of Pfizer Inc, NY, NY 10017

3 0069-3230-66 2
6505-01-137-4628
05-4300-00-5
MADE IN USA
1292

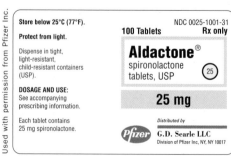
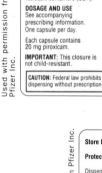

Used with permission from Pfizer Inc.

Store below 25°C (77°F).
Protect from light.
Dispense in tight, light-resistant, child-resistant containers (USP).
DOSAGE AND USE:
See accompanying prescribing information.
Each tablet contains 25 mg spironolactone.

NDC 0025-1001-31
100 Tablets   **Rx only**
Aldactone®
spironolactone tablets, USP   25
25 mg
Distributed by
Pfizer G.D. Searle LLC
Division of Pfizer Inc, NY, NY 10017

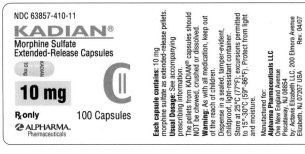

Used with permission of ALPHARMA LLC

NDC 63857-410-11

KADIAN®

Morphine Sulfate
Extended-Release Capsules

10 mg

℞ only   100 Capsules

ALPHARMA.
Pharmaceuticals

Each capsule contains: 10 mg
morphine sulfate as extended-release pellets.
Usual Dosage: See accompanying
prescribing information.
The pellets from KADIAN® capsules should
NOT be chewed, crushed or dissolved.
Warning: As with all medication, keep out
of the reach of children.
Dispense in a sealed, tamper-evident,
childproof, light-resistant container.
Store at 25°C (77°F); excursions permitted
to 15°-30°C (59°-86°F). Protect from light
and moisture.

Manufactured for:
Alpharma Pharmaceuticals LLC
One New England Avenue
Piscataway, NJ 08854
by: Actavis Elizabeth LLC, 200 Elmora Avenue
Elizabeth, NJ 07207 USA   Rev. 04/07

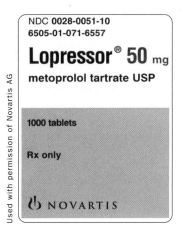

Used with permission of Novartis AG

NDC 0028-0051-10
6505-01-071-6557

Lopressor® 50 mg

metoprolol tartrate USP

1000 tablets

Rx only

Ɖ NOVARTIS

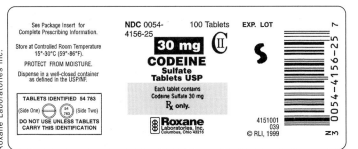

Used with permission of Roxane Laboratories Inc.

See Package Insert for
Complete Prescribing Information.

Store at Controlled Room Temperature
15°-30°C (59°-86°F).

PROTECT FROM MOISTURE.

Dispense in a well-closed container
as defined in the USP/NF.

TABLETS IDENTIFIED 54 783
(Side One)   (Side Two)
**DO NOT USE UNLESS TABLETS
CARRY THIS IDENTIFICATION**

NDC 0054-
4156-25   100 Tablets   EXP. LOT

30 mg ℂ
CODEINE
Sulfate
Tablets USP

Each tablet contains
Codeine Sulfate 30 mg
℞ only.

Roxane
Laboratories, Inc.
Columbus, Ohio 43216

4151001
039
© RLI, 1999

3 0054-4156-25 7

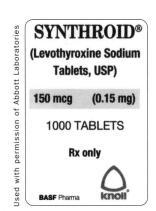

Used with permission of Abbott Laboratories

SYNTHROID®

**(Levothyroxine Sodium
Tablets, USP)**

150 mcg   (0.15 mg)

1000 TABLETS

Rx only

BASF Pharma   **knoll**

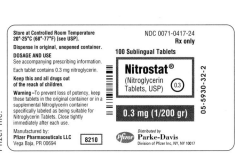

Used with permission from Pfizer Inc.

Store at Controlled Room Temperature
20°-25°C (68°-77°F) [see USP].

Dispense in original, unopened container.

DOSAGE AND USE
See accompanying prescribing information.

Each tablet contains 0.3 mg nitroglycerin.

**Keep this and all drugs out
of the reach of children.**

Warning—To prevent loss of potency, keep
these tablets in the original container or in a
supplemental Nitroglycerin container
specifically labeled as being suitable for
Nitroglycerin Tablets. Close tightly
immediately after each use.

Manufactured by:
Pfizer Pharmaceuticals LLC
Vega Baja, PR 00694   8210

NDC 0071-0417-24
Rx only

100 Sublingual Tablets

Nitrostat®
(Nitroglycerin
Tablets, USP)   0.3

0.3 mg (1/200 gr)

05-5930-32-2

Distributed by
Parke-Davis
Division of Pfizer Inc, NY, NY 10017

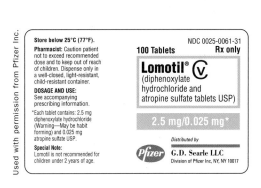

Used with permission from Pfizer Inc.

Store below 25°C (77°F).

Pharmacist: Caution patient
not to exceed recommended
dose and to keep out of reach
of children. Dispense only in
a well-closed, light-resistant,
child-resistant container.

DOSAGE AND USE:
See accompanying
prescribing information.

*Each tablet contains: 2.5 mg
diphenoxylate hydrochloride
(Warning—May be habit
forming) and 0.025 mg
atropine sulfate USP.

Special Note:
Lomotil is not recommended for
children under 2 years of age.

100 Tablets   Rx only   NDC 0025-0061-31

Lomotil® Ⓥ
(diphenoxylate
hydrochloride and
atropine sulfate tablets USP)

2.5 mg/0.025 mg*

Distributed by
G.D. Searle LLC
Division of Pfizer Inc, NY, NY 10017

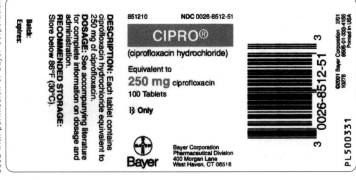

Used with permission of Bayer Corporation

Batch:
Expires:

Store below 86°F (30°C).
RECOMMENDED STORAGE:
administration.
for complete information on dosage and
DOSAGE: See accompanying literature
250 mg of ciprofloxacin.
ciprofloxacin hydrochloride equivalent to
DESCRIPTION: Each tablet contains

851210   NDC 0026-8512-51

CIPRO®
(ciprofloxacin hydrochloride)

Equivalent to
250 mg ciprofloxacin
100 Tablets
℞ Only

©2001 Bayer Corporation
6505-01-338-4195
Printed in USA
10276

Bayer
Bayer Corporation
Pharmaceutical Division
400 Morgan Lane
West Haven, CT 06516

3 0026-8512-51 3

PL500331

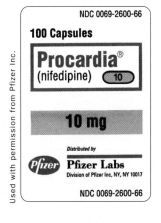

Used with permission from Pfizer Inc.

NDC 0069-2600-66

100 Capsules

Procardia®
(nifedipine)   10

10 mg

Distributed by
Pfizer **Pfizer Labs**
Division of Pfizer Inc, NY, NY 10017

NDC 0069-2600-66

PART IV

30. cefaclor susp. 0.25 g   _____

31. propanolol hydrocloride 120 mg   _____

32. metronidazole 0.75 g   _____

33. piroxicam 40 mg   _____

34. Lopid® 300 mg   _____

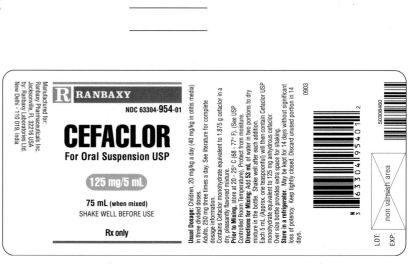

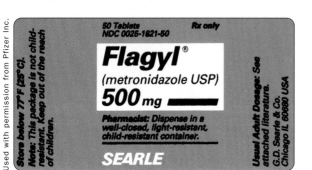

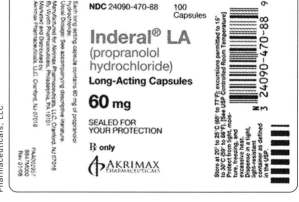

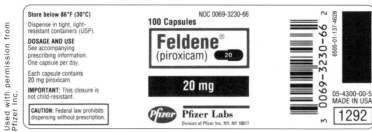

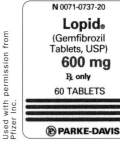

PART V

35. Vantin® 150 mg   _____

36. spironolactone 0.1 g   _____

37. cefpodoxime proxetil 0.2 g   _____

38. Azulfidine® 0.75 g   _____

39. potassium chloride 40 mEq   _____

40. Cipro® 250 mg   _____

Used with permission of Pharmaceutical Associates, Inc.

Delivers **15 mL**
NDC 0121-0465-15
POTASSIUM CHLORIDE
ORAL SOLUTION USP 10%
20 mEq per 15 mL
Sugar Free   Alcohol 5%
DILUTE BEFORE USING

(01) 0 03 01210 46515 4
Rx ONLY
FOR INSTITUTIONAL USE ONLY
PHARMACEUTICAL ASSOCIATES, INC.
GREENVILLE, SC 29605
SEE INSERT

Used with permission from Pfizer Inc.

Store below 25°C (77°F).
Protect from light.
Dispense in tight,
light-resistant,
child-resistant containers
(USP).
DOSAGE AND USE:
See accompanying
prescribing information.
Each tablet contains 100 mg
spironolactone.

NDC 0025-1031-31
Rx only

100 Tablets

Aldactone®
spironolactone
tablets, USP   (100)

100 mg

Distributed by

Pfizer **G.D. Searle LLC**
Division of Pfizer Inc, NY, NY 10017

2137

N3 0025-1031-31 1
05-6589-32-1

Used with permission of Pfizer Inc.

Azulfidine®
sulfasalazine tablets, USP

500 mg

Rx only

MADE IN SWEDEN

Mfd. for: Pharmacia & Upjohn Co.
Kalamazoo, MI 49001, USA
by: Pharmacia & Upjohn AB
Stockholm, Sweden

300 Tablets

**Pharmacia
&Upjohn**

Used with permission of Pfizer Inc.

NDC 0009-3615-03
50 mL (when mixed)

Vantin® For Oral Suspension

cefpodoxime proxetil
for oral suspension

100 mg per 5 mL

Equivalent to 100 mg per 5 mL
cefpodoxime when constituted

**Pharmacia
&Upjohn**

Used with permission of Bayer Corporation

851210   NDC 0026-8512-51

Batch:
Expires:

DESCRIPTION: Each tablet contains
ciprofloxacin hydrochloride equivalent to
250 mg of ciprofloxacin.
DOSAGE: See accompanying literature
for complete information on dosage and
administration.
RECOMMENDED STORAGE:
Store below 86°F (30°C).

CIPRO®
(ciprofloxacin hydrochloride)

Equivalent to
250 mg ciprofloxacin
100 Tablets

Rx Only

Bayer   Bayer Corporation
Pharmaceutical Division
400 Morgan Lane
West Haven, CT 06516

©2001 Bayer Corporation   2101
10276   6505-01-353-4195
Printed in USA

3 0026-8512-51 3
PL500331

Answers

1. 3 tab	**9.** 3 tab	**18.** 2 cap	**27.** 2 tab	**36.** 1 tab
2. 2 tab	**10.** 2 cap	**19.** 1½ tab	**28.** 1½ tab	**37.** 10 mL
3. 2 cap	**11.** 2 tab	**20.** 3 tab	**29.** 2 tab	**38.** 1½ tab
4. 2 cap	**12.** 2 tab	**21.** 1 cap	**30.** 10 mL	**39.** 30 mL
5. 1 cap	**13.** 2 tab	**22.** 1 cap	**31.** 2 cap	**40.** 1 tab
6. 10 mL	**14.** 2 tab	**23.** 2 cap	**32.** 1½ tab	
7. 2 tab	**15.** 2 tab	**24.** 1 tab	**33.** 2 cap	
8. 1 tab	**16.** 3 tab	**25.** 3 cap	**34.** ½ tab	
	17. 2 tab	**26.** 1½ tab	**35.** 7.5 mL	

HYPODERMIC SYRINGE MEASUREMENT

A variety of hypodermic syringes is in clinical use. This chapter focuses most heavily on the frequently used 3 mL syringe. However, larger volume syringes are used on occasion, so it is necessary that you learn the **differences** as well as the **similarities** of all syringes in use.

Regardless of a syringe's volume or capacity—0.5, 1, 3, 5, 10, or 20 mL— all except specialized insulin syringes **are calibrated in mL**. Because some syringe manufacturers have not yet replaced the labeling on their syringes with the official mL volume measurement, you may still see cc on syringes. Keep in mind, however, that these two measures, mL and cc, are essentially identical. They will be correctly referred to throughout this text as mL. The various capacity syringes contain **calibrations that differ from each other**. Recognizing the difference in syringe calibrations is the chief safety concern of this chapter.

 The calibrations on different volume syringes differ from each other, requiring particular care in dosage measurement.

Objectives

The learner will measure parenteral solutions using:

1. a standard 3 mL syringe.
2. a tuberculin syringe.
3. 5 and 10 mL syringes.
4. a 20 mL syringe.

STANDARD 3 mL SYRINGE

The most commonly used hypodermic syringe is the 3 mL size illustrated in Figure 8-1. Notice the calibrations for the metric mL scale, and that **longer calibrations** identify zero (0) and each ½ and full mL measure. These longer calibrations are numbered: ½, 1, 1½, 2, 2½, and 3.

Next, notice the **number of calibrations in each mL**, which is **10**, indicating that on this syringe, each mL is **calibrated in tenths**. Tenths of a mL are written as **decimal fractions**; for example 1.2 mL, 2.5 mL, or 0.4 mL. Also, notice the arrow on this syringe, which identifies a 0.8 mL dosage.

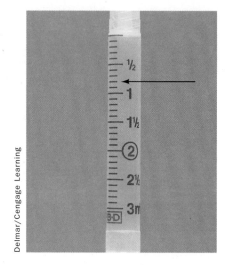

Figure 8-1 | A 3 mL syringe.

Problems 8.1

Use decimal numbers—for example, 2.2 mL—to identify the measurements
indicated by the arrows on the standard 3 mL syringes that follow.

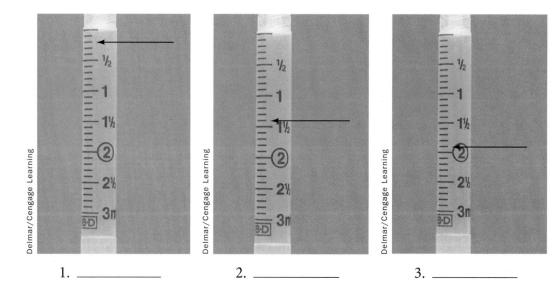

1. _____

2. _____

3. _____

Answers   1. 0.2 mL   **2.** 1.4 mL   **3.** 1.9 mL

Did you have difficulty with the 0.2 mL calibration in Problem 1? Remember that
the first long calibration on all syringes is zero. It is slightly longer than the 0.1 mL
and subsequent one-tenth calibrations. Be careful not to mistakenly count it as 0.1 mL.

You have just been looking at photos of syringe barrels only. In assembled
syringes, the colored suction tip of the plunger has two widened areas in contact
with the barrel that look like two distinct rings. **Calibrations are read from the
front, or top, ring.** Do not become confused by the second, or bottom, ring or by
the raised middle section of the suction tip.

Problems 8.2

What dosages are measured by the following three assembled syringes?

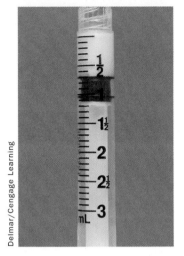

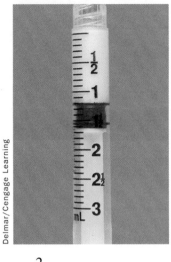

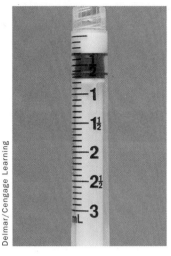

1. _____   2. _____   3. _____

Answers 1. 0.7 mL **2.** 1.2 mL **3.** 0.3 mL

Problems 8.3

Draw an arrow or shade in the following syringe barrels to indicate the required dosages. Have your instructor check your accuracy.

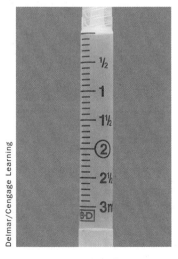

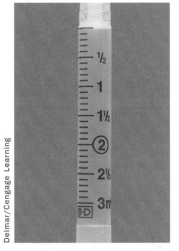

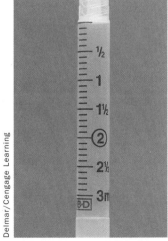

1. 1.3 mL   2. 2.4 mL   3. 0.9 mL

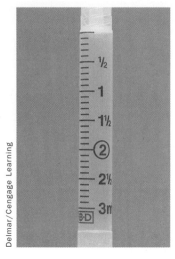

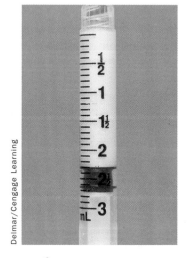

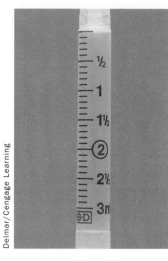

4. 2.5 mL

5. 1.7 mL

6. 2.1 mL

Verify your answers with your instructor.

Problems 8.4

Identify the dosages measured on the following 3 mL syringes.

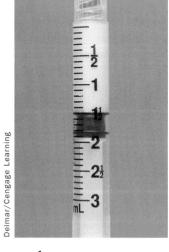

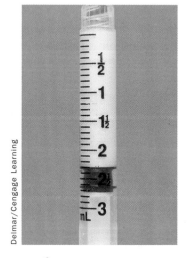

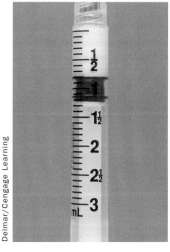

1. _____

2. _____

3. _____

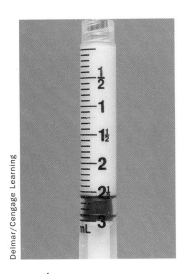

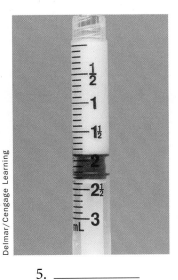

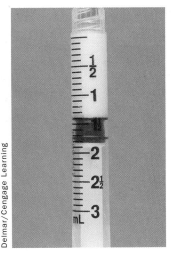

4. _____

5. _____

6. _____

SAFETY SYRINGES

A number of safety syringes has been developed in recent years to reduce the danger of accidental contaminated needle sticks. Several of these syringes are illustrated in the following photos. Take a few minutes to become familiar with them, as you will in all probability be using them in the clinical setting.

Refer first to the photos in Figure 8-2, which show two B-D SafetyGlide™ syringes. Each of these syringes contains a protective needle guard that can be activated by a single finger to cover and seal the needle after injection.

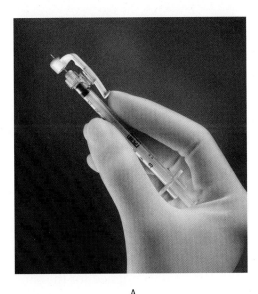

A

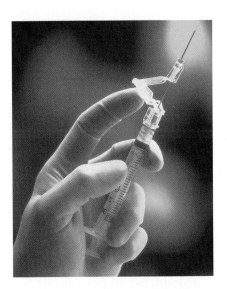

B

Figure 8-2A and B | SafetyGlide™ syringes. Courtesy and © Becton, Dickinson and Company.

The syringe shown in Figure 8-3, the VanishPoint®, has a needle that automatically retracts into the barrel after injection.

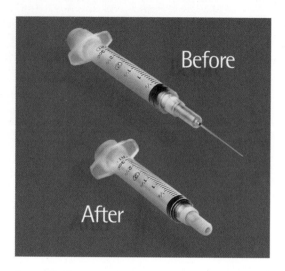

Figure 8-3 | VanishPoint®. Courtesy of Retractable Technologies.

A third type of safety needle commonly used is the Magellan Safety Needle by Covidien™, as shown in Figure 8-4. This design also offers one-handed activation. It can be activated one of three ways: by thumb, forefinger, or on a flat surface. As with the other safety syringes, once activated, its safety shield covers the entire needle, providing protection during and after disposal.

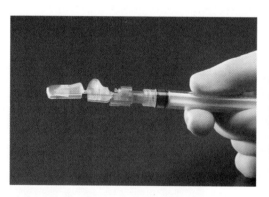
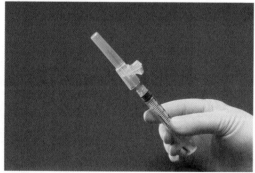

A   B

Figure 8-4A and B | Magellan Safety Needle. Courtesy of Covidien.

TUBERCULIN (TB) SYRINGE

When very small dosages are required, they are measured in special tuberculin (TB) **0.5 or 1 mL syringes calibrated in hundredths**. Originally designed for the small dosages required for tuberculin skin testing, these syringes are also widely used in a variety of sensitivity and allergy tests. Pediatric dosages frequently require measurement in hundredths, as does heparin, an anticoagulant drug.

Refer to the 0.5 mL TB syringe in Figure 8-5, and take a careful look at its metric calibrated hundredth scale. Notice that slightly longer calibrations identify zero, 0.05, 0.1, 0.15, 0.2, and so on through the 0.5 mL measure. Shorter calibrations lie between these to measure the hundredths. Each tenth mL, .1, .2, .3, .4, and .5, is numbered on this particular TB syringe. Take a moment to study the dosage measured by the arrow in Figure 8-5, which is 0.43 mL.

The closeness and small size of TB syringe calibrations mandate particular care and an unhurried approach in TB syringe dosage measurement.

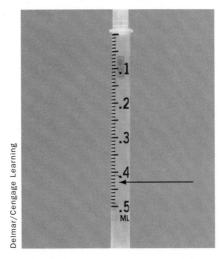

Figure 8-5 | A tuberculin (TB) syringe.

Problems 8.5

Identify the measurements on the six TB syringes provided.

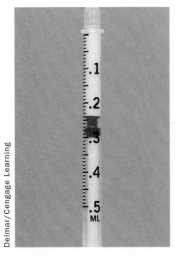

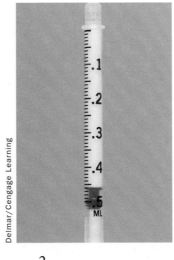

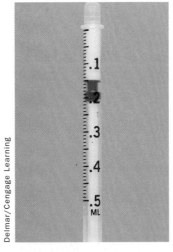

1. _____   2. _____   3. _____

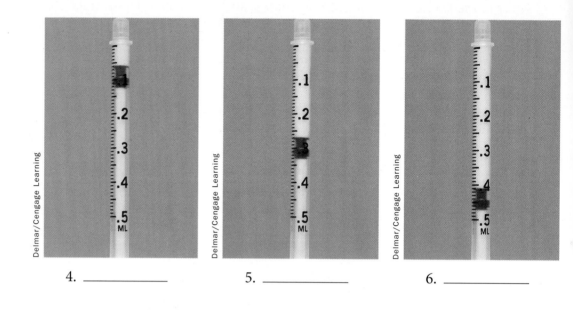

4. _____   5. _____   6. _____

Answers **1.** 0.24 mL **2.** 0.46 mL **3.** 0.15 mL **4.** 0.06 mL **5.** 0.27 mL **6.** 0.41 mL

Problems 8.6

Draw an arrow on the barrel to identify the dosages indicated on these TB syringes. Have your instructor check your answers.

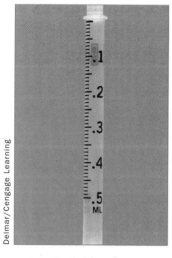

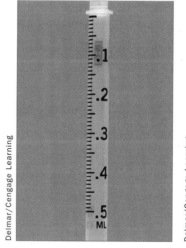

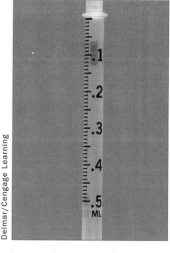

1. 0.28 mL   2. 0.32 mL   3. 0.45 mL

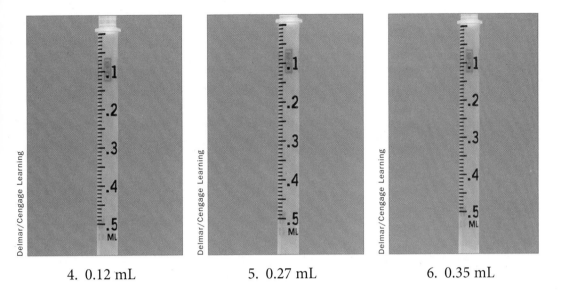

4. 0.12 mL   5. 0.27 mL   6. 0.35 mL

Verify your answers with your instructor.

5 AND 10 mL SYRINGES

When volumes larger than 3 mL are required, a 5 or 10 mL syringe is typically used. Refer to Figure 8-6, and examine the calibrations between the numbered mLs to determine how these syringes are calibrated.

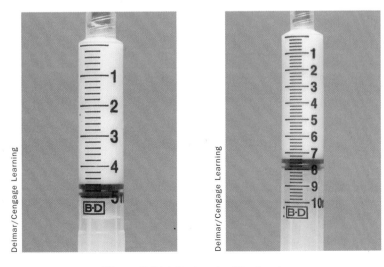

Figure 8-6 | A 5 mL and a 10 mL syringe.

As you may have discovered, the calibrations divide each mL of these syringes into **five** so that **each shorter calibration actually measures 0.2 mL**. The 5 mL syringe on the left measures 4.6 mL, and the 10 mL syringe on the right measures 7.4 mL. These syringes are most often used to measure whole rather than fractional dosages, but in your practice readings, we will include a full range of measurements.

Problems 8.7

What dosages are measured on the following syringes?

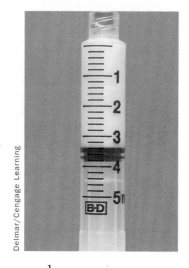

1. _____

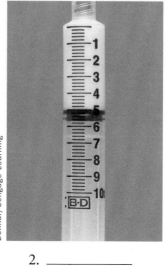

2. _____

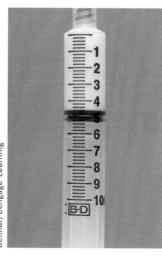

3. _____

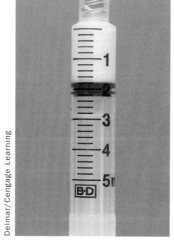

4. _____

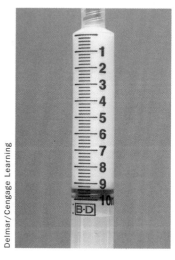

5. _____

Answers **1.** 3.4 mL **2.** 5 mL **3.** 4.6 mL **4.** 1.8 mL **5.** 9.4 mL

Problems 8.8

Measure the dosages indicated on the syringes provided. Have an instructor check your accuracy.

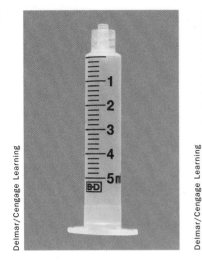

1. 1.4 mL

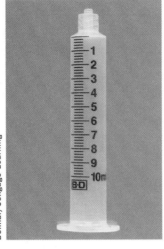

2. 3.2 mL

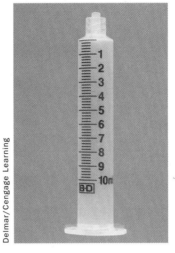

3. 6.8 mL

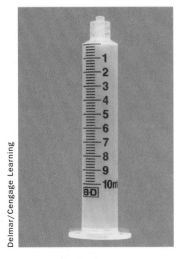

4. 9.4 mL

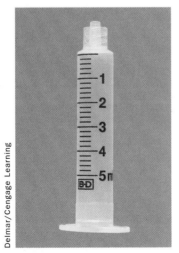

5. 4.4 mL

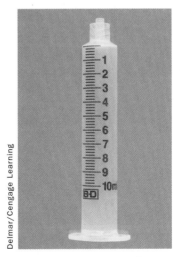

6. 5.6 mL

Verify your answers with your instructor.

20 mL AND LARGER SYRINGES

Examine the 20 mL syringe in Figure 8-7, and determine how it is calibrated.

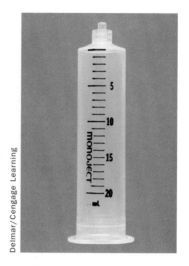

Figure 8-7 | A 20 mL syringe.

As you can see, this syringe is calibrated in **1 mL increments**, with longer calibrations identifying the 0, 5, 10, 15, and 20 mL volumes. Syringes with a capacity larger than 20 mL are also calibrated in full mL measures. These syringes are used only for measurement of very large volumes.

Problems 8.9

What dosages are measured on these syringes?

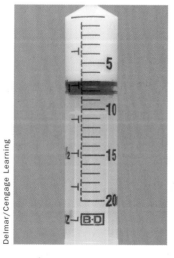

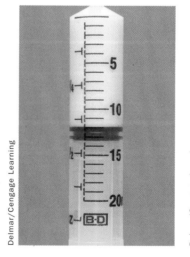

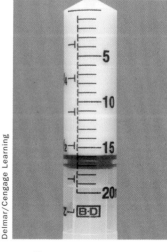

1. _____   2. _____   3. _____

Answers   1. 7 mL   **2.** 12 mL   **3.** 16 mL

Problems 8.10

Shade in or draw arrows on the three syringe barrels provided to identify the volumes listed. Have your answers checked by your instructor.

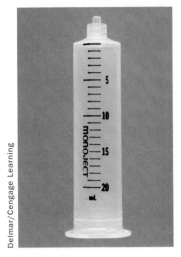

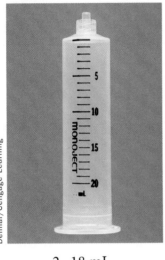

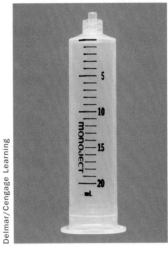

1. 11 mL

2. 18 mL

3. 9 mL

Verify your answers with your instructor.

Summary

This concludes your introduction to syringe calibrations. The important points to remember from this chapter are:

- 3 mL syringes are calibrated in tenths.

- TB syringes are calibrated in hundredths.

- 5 and 10 mL syringes are calibrated in fifths (two-tenths).

- Syringes larger than 10 mL are calibrated in full mL measures.

- The first long calibration on all syringes indicates zero.

- All syringe calibrations must be read from the top, or front, ring of the plunger's suction tip.

Summary Self-Test

Identify the dosages measured on the following syringes

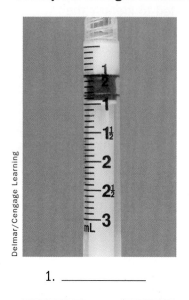

1. _____

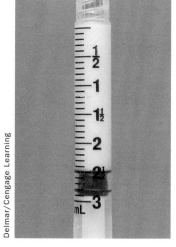

2. _____

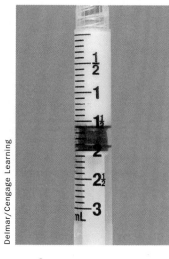

3. _____

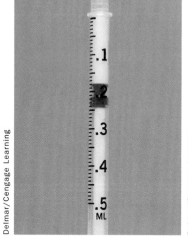

4. _____

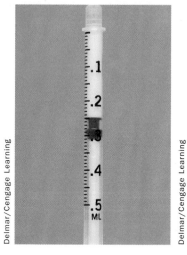

5. _____

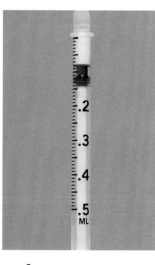

6. _____

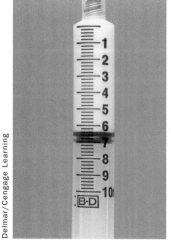

7. _____

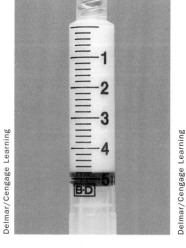

8. _____

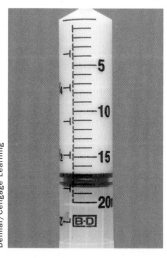

9. _____

Draw arrows or shade the barrels on the following syringes/cartridges to measure the indicated dosages. Have your answers checked by your instructor.

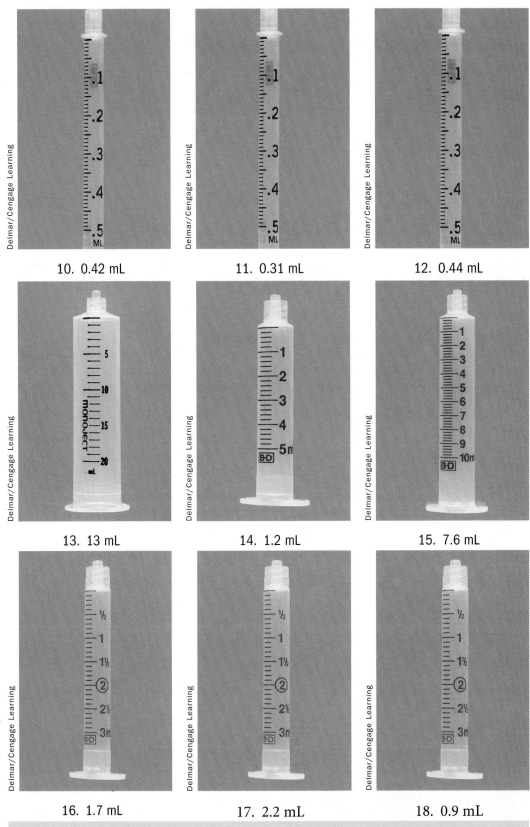

10. 0.42 mL

11. 0.31 mL

12. 0.44 mL

13. 13 mL

14. 1.2 mL

15. 7.6 mL

16. 1.7 mL

17. 2.2 mL

18. 0.9 mL

Answers   **1.** 0.5 mL   **2.** 2.5 mL   **3.** 1.6 mL   **4.** 0.18 mL   **5.** 0.25 mL   **6.** 0.08 mL   **7.** 6.4 mL   **8.** 4.8 mL   **9.** 17 mL   **10–18.** Verify your answers with your instructor.

PARENTERAL MEDICATION LABELS AND DOSAGE CALCULATION

Objectives

The learner will:

1. read parenteral solution labels and identify dosage strengths.

2. calculate average parenteral dosages from the labels provided.

3. measure parenteral dosages in metric, milliequivalent, unit, percentage, and ratio strengths using 3 mL, TB, 5, 10, and 20 mL syringes.

Parenteral medications are administered by injection, with intravenous (IV), intramuscular (IM), and subcutaneous (subcut) being the most frequently used routes. The labels of oral and parenteral solutions are very similar, but the size of the average parenteral dosage label is much smaller. Intramuscular solutions are manufactured so that the **average adult dosage will be contained in a volume of between 0.5 mL and 3 mL**, with subcutaneous injections being smaller, and seldom exceeding 1 mL. Excessively larger or smaller volumes would need to be questioned and calculations rechecked.

 Volumes larger than 3 mL are difficult for a single IM injection site to absorb, and the 0.5 to 3 mL volume can be used as a guideline for accuracy of calculations in IM and subcutaneous dosages

Intravenous medication administration is usually a two-step procedure. The dosage is prepared first, then may be further diluted in IV fluids before administration. In this chapter, we will be concerned only with the **first step of IV drug preparation, which is accurate measurement of the prescribed dosage**.

Parenteral medications are packaged in a variety of single-use glass ampules, single- and multiple-use rubber-stoppered vials, and premeasured syringes and cartridges. See Figure 9-1.

READING METRIC/SI SOLUTION LABELS

Let's begin by looking at parenteral solution labels on which the dosages are expressed in metric units of measure.

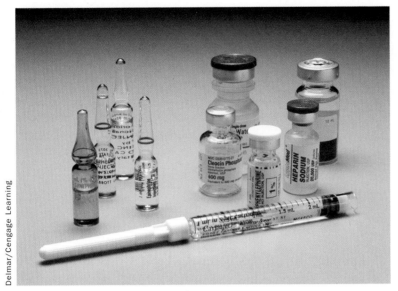

Figure 9-1 | Ampules, vials, and a pre-filled cartridge.

Delmar/Cengage Learning

EXAMPLE 1

Refer to the Vistaril® label in Figure 9-2. The immediate difference you will notice between this and oral solution labels is the **size**. Ampules and vials are small and their labels are small, which requires that they be **read with particular care**. The information, however, is similar to oral labels. Vistaril is the trade name of the drug; hydroxyzine hydrochloride is the generic name. The dosage strength is 50 mg per mL (in the red rectangular area). The total vial contents are 10 mL (in black, center). Keep in mind that average intramuscular and subcutaneous dosages usually consist of one-half to double the average dosage strength, which for this IM Vistaril is 50 mg per mL.

> For 50 mg, you would give 1 mL
> For 25 mg, you would give 0.5 mL
> For 100 mg, you would give 2 mL
> For 75 mg, you would give 1.5 mL

These average dosages are within the usual 0.5 to 3 mL IM volume.

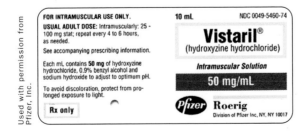

Used with permission from Pfizer, Inc.

Figure 9-2

Figure 9-3

EXAMPLE 2

The Robinul® (glycopyrrolate) medication in Figure 9-3 has a dosage strength of 0.2 mg/mL.

> For a 0.2 mg dosage, you would give 1 mL
> For a 0.1 mg dosage, you would give 0.5 mL
> For a 200 mcg dosage, you would give 1 mL
> For a 100 mcg dosage, you would give 0.5 mL
> For a 0.4 mg dosage, you would give 2 mL
> For a 400 mcg dosage, you would give 2 mL

Problems 9.1

Refer to the Celestone® label in Figure 9-4 to answer the following questions.

1. What is the dosage strength of this solution?   _____
2. How many mL are required for a dosage of 3 mg?   _____
3. How many mL for a 6 mg dosage?   _____
4. How many mL for a 9 mg dosage?   _____
5. How many mL for a 12 mg dosage?   _____

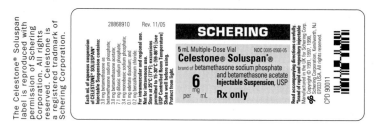

Figure 9-4

Answers   **1.** 6 mg/mL   **2.** 0.5 mL   **3.** 1 mL   **4.** 1.5 mL   **5.** 2 mL

Problems 9.2

Refer to the gentamicin label in Figure 9-5 to answer the following questions.

1. What is the total volume of this vial? _____

2. What is the dosage strength? _____

3. If 80 mg were ordered, how many mL would this be? _____

4. If 60 mg were ordered, how many mL would this be? _____

5. How many mL would you need to prepare a 20 mg dosage? _____

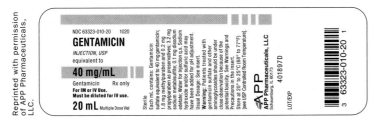

Figure 9-5

Answers   1. 20 mL   **2.** 40 mg/mL   **3.** 2 mL   **4.** 1.5 mL   **5.** 0.5 mL

PERCENT (%) AND RATIO SOLUTION LABELS

Drugs labeled as **percentage solutions** often express the dosage strength in **metric measures in addition to percentage strength**. The lidocaine label in Figure 9-6, a 2% solution, is an example.

But directly underneath this is a "20 mg/mL" designation. Lidocaine HCl is most often ordered in mg, but it is also used as a local anesthetic, and when it is, a physician may ask you to prepare a volume dosage specifying % strength.

Problems 9.3

Refer to the lidocaine label in Figure 9-6 to answer the following questions.

1. How many mL are needed for a 10 mg dosage? _____

2. How many mL for a 20 mg dosage? _____

3. If you are asked to prepare 5 mL of a 2% solution? _____

4. If you are asked to prepare 15 mg? _____

NDC 10019-019-57

Lidocaine **2%**
HCl Injection, USP

(20 mg/mL)   ℞ only
FOR INFILTRATION AND NERVE BLOCK
NOT FOR SPINAL OR EPIDURAL ANESTHESIA
50 mL Multiple Dose Vial

Baxter   **eSi LEDERLE™**
Mfd. for **Baxter Healthcare Corporation** affiliate
by: Elkins-Sinn, Cherry Hill, NJ 08003   400-747-01

Each mL contains lidocaine hydrochloride 20 mg, sodium chloride 6 mg
and methylparaben 1 mg in Water for
Injection. pH 5.0-7.0; sodium hydroxide and/or hydrochloric acid used,
if needed, for pH adjustment.

Usual Dosage: See package insert for
complete prescribing information.

Store at controlled room temperature
15°-30°C (59°-86°F).

Copyright Baxter International Inc.

Figure 9-6

Problems 9.4

Refer to the lidocaine label in Figure 9-7 to answer the following questions.

1. What is the percentage strength of this lidocaine solution?   _____

2. How many mL does the vial contain?   _____

3. If you are asked to prepare 20 mL of a 1% lidocaine solution, how many mL will you draw up in the syringe?   _____

4. What is the metric dosage strength of this solution?   _____

5. If you are asked to prepare 25 mg from this vial, what volume will you draw up?   _____

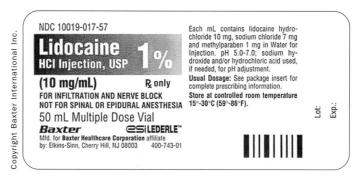

Figure 9-7

Refer to the calcium gluconate label in Figure 9-8 to answer the following questions.

6. What is the percentage strength of this solution?   _____

7. How many mL does this preparation contain?   _____

8. What is the per mL mEq dosage strength of this solution?   _____

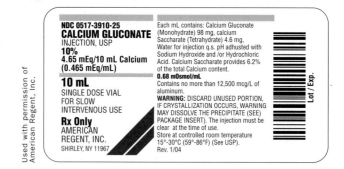

Figure 9-8

Parenteral medications expressed in **ratio strengths** are not common, and **when they are ordered, it will be by number of mL**. Ratio labels may also contain dosages in metric weights.

Problems 9.5

Refer to the epinephrine label in Figure 9-9 to answer the following questions.

1. What is the ratio strength of this solution?   _____

2. What volume is this contained in?   _____

3. What is the metric dosage strength of this solution?   _____

NDC 0517-1071-25
EPINEPHRINE
INJECTION, USP **1:1000** (1 mg/mL)

1 mL AMPULE
FOR SC AND IM USE. FOR IV
AND IC USE AFTER DILUTION.
Rx Only
CONTAINS NO SULFITES.
PRESERVATIVE FREE.
Store at controlled room temperature
up to 25°C (77°F) (See USP).   Rev. 1/04
AMERICAN REGENT, INC.
SHIRLEY, NY 11967

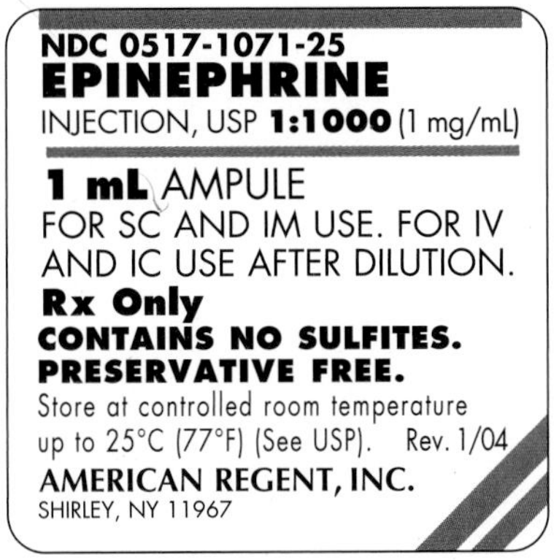

Used with permission from American Regent, Inc.

Figure 9-9

Answers   1. 1 : 1000   **2.** 1 mL   **3.** 1 mg/mL

SOLUTIONS MEASURED IN INTERNATIONAL UNITS

A number of drugs are measured in **International Units**. The following labels will introduce you to several examples.

Problems 9.6

Refer to the heparin label in Figure 9-10 to answer the following questions.

1. What is the total volume of this vial?   _____

2. What is the dosage strength?   _____

3. If a volume of 1.5 mL is prepared, how many units will this be?   _____

4. How many mL will you need to prepare a dosage of 5500 units?   _____

5. If 0.25 mL of this medication is prepared, what dosage will this be?   _____

NDC 0025-6589-82
HEPARIN SODIUM
Injection, USP
1,000 units/mL
Derived from porcine intestinal mucosa
For intravenous or subcutaneous use
10mL
Multiple Dose Vial   Rx only

Sterile, nonpyrogenic.
Each mL contains: 1,000 USP units
heparin sodium; 9 mg sodium
chloride; 0.15% methylparaben;
0.015% propylparaben; water for
injection q.s. Made isotonic with
sodium chloride. Hydrochloric acid
and/or sodium hydroxide may have
been added for pH adjustment.

Use only if solution is clear
and seal is intact.

Store at 25°C (77°F);
excursions permitted to 15° to 30°C
(59° to 86°F).

SL SIMULATED LABEL For Educational Purposes Only

354588-23

Delmar/Cengage Learning

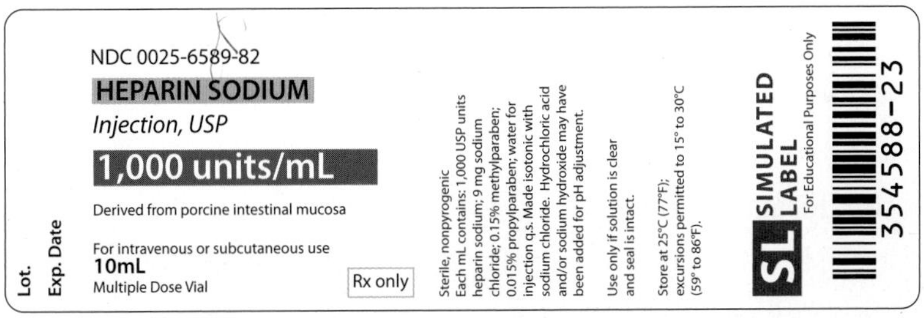

Lot.   Exp. Date

Figure 9-10

Refer to the Bicillin® C-R label in Figure 9-11 to answer the following questions.

6. What is the dosage strength of this medication?   _____

7. If 600,000 units are ordered, how many mL would
   this require?   _____

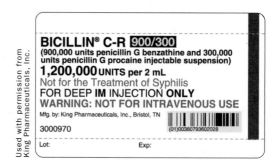

Figure 9-11

Answers   1. 10 mL   **2.** 1000 units/mL   **3.** 1500 units   **4.** 5.5 mL   **5.** 250 units
6. 1,200,000 units/2 mL   **7.** 1 mL

SOLUTIONS MEASURED AS MILLIEQUIVALENTS (mEq)

The next four labels will introduce you to milliequivalent (mEq) dosages. Refer to the calcium gluconate label in Figure 9-12 and notice that in addition to its 10% strength, this vial has a dosage of 0.465 mEq/mL. If a dosage of 0.465 mEq were ordered, you would draw up 1 mL in the syringe.

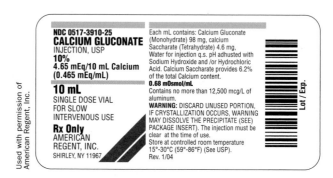

Figure 9-12

Problems 9.7

Refer to the potassium chloride label in Figure 9-13 to answer the following questions.

1. What are the total dosage and volume of this vial?   _____

2. What is the dosage in mEq per mL?   _____

3. If you were asked to prepare 15 mEq for addition to an IV,
   what volume would you draw up?   _____

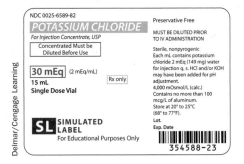

Figure 9-13

Refer to the potassium acetate label in Figure 9-14 to answer the following dosage questions.

4. What is the strength of this solution in mEq per mL?   _____

5. If you were asked to prepare 40 mEq for addition to an IV solution, what volume would you draw up in the syringe?   _____

6. What volume would you need for a dosage of 20 mEq?   _____

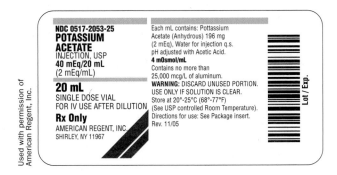

Figure 9-14

Refer to the sodium bicarbonate label in Figure 9-15. Notice that this solution lists the drug strength in mEq, percentage, and g. Read the label very carefully to answer the following questions.

7. What is the dosage strength expressed in mEq/mL?   _____

8. What is the total volume of the vial, and how many mEq does this volume contain?   _____

9. What is the strength per mL expressed as g?   _____

10. If you were asked to prepare 10 mL of an 8.4% sodium bicarbonate solution, what volume would you draw up in a syringe?   _____

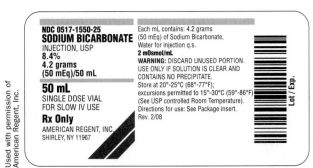

Figure 9-15

Summary

This concludes the introduction to parenteral solution labels. The important points to remember from this chapter are:

- The most commonly used parenteral administration routes are IV, IM, and subcutaneous.

- The labels of most parenteral solutions are quite small and must be read with particular care.

- The average IM dosage will be contained in a volume of between 0.5 mL and 3 mL.

- These 0.5 to 3 mL volumes can be used as a guideline to accuracy of calculations.

- The average subcutaneous dosage volume is between 0.5 and 1 mL.

- IV medication preparation is usually a two-step procedure: measurement of the dosage, then dilution according to manufacturers' recommendations or a physician's or prescriber's order.

- Parenteral drugs may be measured in metric, ratio, percentage, unit, or mEq dosages.

- If dosages are ordered by percentage or ratio strength, they are usually specified in mL to be administered.

- Most IM dosages are prepared using a 3 mL syringe.

- Most subcutaneous dosages are prepared using a 3 mL or tuberculin syringe.

Summary Self-Test

Read the parenteral drug labels provided to measure the following dosages. Then, indicate on the syringe provided exactly how much solution you will draw up to obtain these dosages. Have your answers checked by your instructor to be sure you have measured the dosages correctly.

Dosage Ordered   **mL Needed**

1. terbutaline sulfate 500 mcg   _____

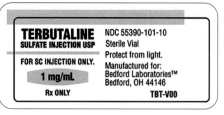

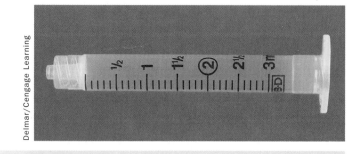

Dosage Ordered

mL Needed

2. furosemide 10 mg

_____

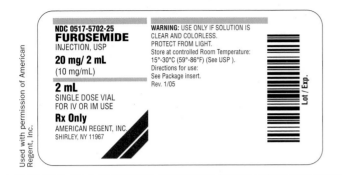

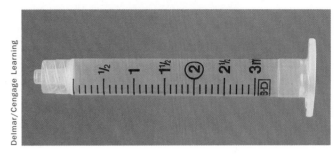

3. heparin 2500 units

_____

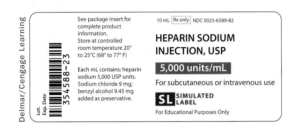

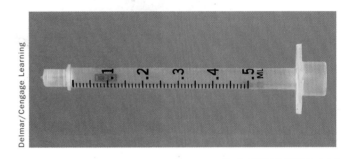

4. acyclovir Na 100 mg

_____

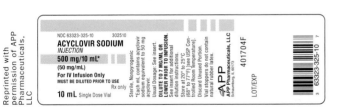

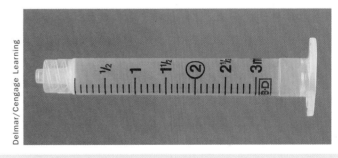

Dosage Ordered	**mL Needed**

5. atropine 0.2 mg

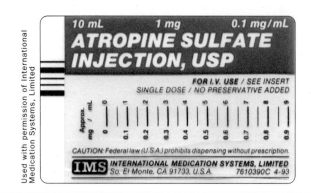

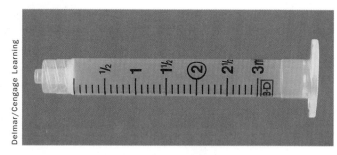

6. hydroxyzine HCl 25 mg

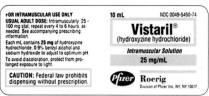

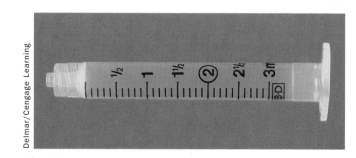

7. Robinul® 100 mcg

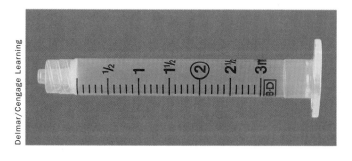

Dosage Ordered

mL Needed

8. nitroglycerine 25 mg

_____

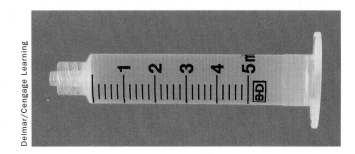

9. methotrexate 0.25 g

_____

10. cyanocobalamin 1 mg

_____

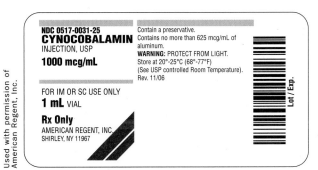

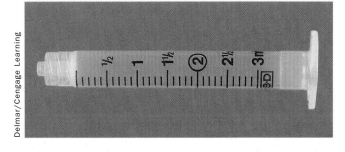

Dosage Ordered   **mL Needed**

11. hydralazine hydrochloride 10 mg   _____

NDC 0517-0901-25
**HYDRALAZINE
HYDROCHLORIDE**
INJECTION, USP
20 mg / mL

1 mL SINGLE DOSE VIAL
FOR IM OR IV USE

Rx Only

AMERICAN REGENT, INC.
SHIRLEY, NY 11967

WARNING: DISCARD UNUSED PORTION. Store at 20°-25°C (68°-77°F) (See USP Controlled Room Temperature). Directions for Use: See Package Insert. Rev. 11/05

12. epinephrine 2 mg   _____

NDC 0517-1071-25
EPINEPHRINE
INJECTION, USP **1:1000** (1 mg/mL)

1 mL AMPULE
FOR SC AND IM USE. FOR IV AND IC USE AFTER DILUTION.
Rx Only
**CONTAINS NO SULFITES.
PRESERVATIVE FREE.**
Store at controlled room temperature up to 25°C (77°F) (See USP).   Rev. 1/04
AMERICAN REGENT, INC.
SHIRLEY, NY 11967

13. Fentanyl® 125 mcg   _____

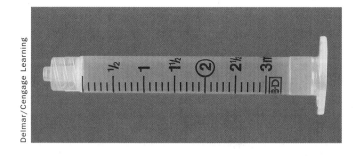

NDC 10019-033-72
Fentanyl
Citrate Injection, USP

C II

R only

250 mcg/5 mL
50 mcg/mL (0.05 mg/mL)
10 x 5 mL DOSETTE® Ampuls
**FOR INTRAVENOUS
OR INTRAMUSCULAR USE**

Each mL contains fentanyl citrate equivalent to 50 mcg (0.05 mg) fentanyl base in Water for Injection. pH 4.0-7.5; sodium hydroxide and/or hydrochloric acid added, if needed, for pH adjustment. Contains no preservative.
Usual Dosage: See package insert for complete prescribing information.
PROTECT FROM LIGHT: Keep covered in carton until time of use.
Store at controlled room temperature 15°-30°C (59°-86°F).
To open ampuls, ignore color line; break at constriction.

Baxter   **≈SiLEDERLE™**
Mfd. for an affiliate of
Baxter Healthcare Corporation
Deerfield, IL 60015 USA
by: Elkins-Sinn, Inc., Cherry Hill, NJ 08003   460-120-00

DOSETTE® is a registered trademark of A.H. Robins Company

Dosage Ordered

mL Needed

14. calcium gluconate 0.93 mEq

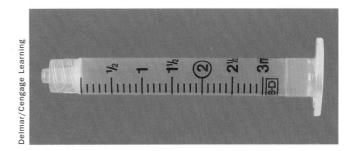

15. Ceftriaxone 0.7 g

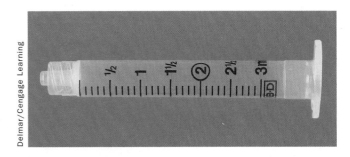

16. heparin 500 units

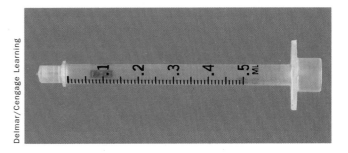

17. ondansetron 3 mg

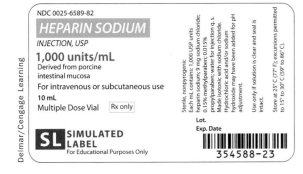

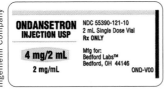

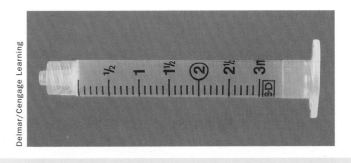

Dosage Ordered   **mL Needed**

18. epinephrine 0.5 mg

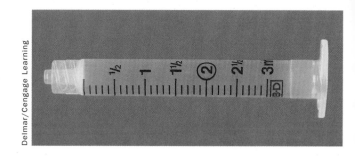

_____

19. Ketorolac tromethamine 30 mg

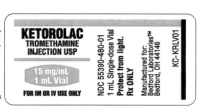

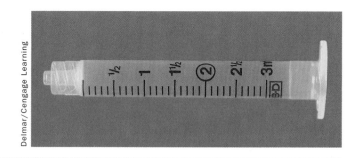

_____

20. gentamicin 60 mg

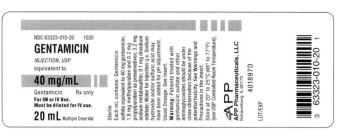

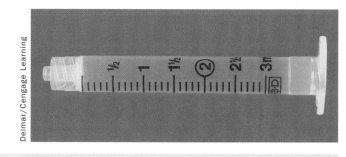

_____

Dosage Ordered

mL Needed

21. lidocaine HCl 50 mg _____

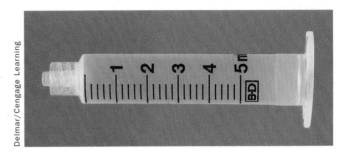

NDC 10019-017-56

Lidocaine **1%**
HCl Injection, USP

(10 mg/mL) R only
FOR INFILTRATION AND NERVE BLOCK
NOT FOR SPINAL OR EPIDURAL ANESTHESIA
30 mL Multiple Dose Vial

Baxter **LEDERLE**™
Mfd. for **Baxter Healthcare Corporation** affiliate
by: Elkins-Sinn, Cherry Hill, NJ 08003   400-741-01

Each mL contains lidocaine hydrochloride 10 mg, sodium chloride 7 mg
and methylparaben 1 mg in Water for
Injection. pH 5.0-7.0; sodium hydroxide and/or hydrochloric acid used,
if needed, for pH adjustment.
Usual Dosage: See package insert for
complete prescribing information.
Store at controlled room temperature
15°-30°C (59°-86°F).

Lot:
Exp.:

Copyright Baxter International Inc.

22. sodium chloride 40 mEq _____

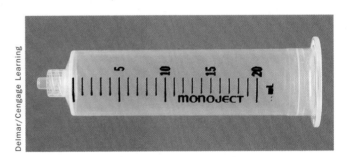

NDC 0025-6589-82

SODIUM CHLORIDE
INJECTION, USP

CONCENTRATED
PHARMACY BULK PACKAGE–
Not for direct infusion

23.4% 4 mEq/mL
FOR IV USE ONLY
AFTER DILUTION

100 mL   Rx only

**SL SIMULATED
LABEL**
For Educational Purposes Only

Preservative Free
Each mL contains: sodium chloride 234 mg;
water for injection q.s. pH may have been
adjusted with hydrochloric acid.

8008 mOsmol/L 4,000 mEq/L
Directions for pharmacy bulk package: Swab
stopper with an antiseptic solution. Withdraw
contents of the vial using a sterile dispensing
set. If prompt fluid transfer is not possible, a
maximum time of 4 hours from the time of
initial entry is allowed to complete the
transferring operations. Discard the container
no later than 4 hours after initial closure.

Use only if solution is clear and seal intact.
Store at controlled room temperature 15° to
30°C (59° to 86°F). Do not freeze.

Lot.
Exp. Date

354588-23

Delmar/Cengage Learning

23. atropine 200 mcg _____

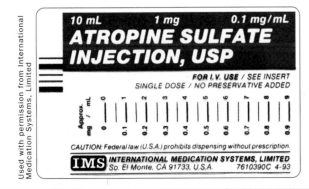

10 mL   **1 mg**   **0.1 mg/mL**
**ATROPINE SULFATE
INJECTION, USP**

FOR I.V. USE */ SEE INSERT*
SINGLE DOSE / NO PRESERVATIVE ADDED

CAUTION: Federal law (U.S.A.) prohibits dispensing without prescription.
IMS INTERNATIONAL MEDICATION SYSTEMS, LIMITED
So. El Monte, CA 91733, U.S.A.   7610390C 4-93

Used with permission from International Medication Systems, Limited

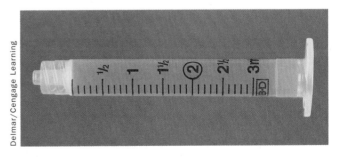

Delmar/Cengage Learning

Dosage Ordered   **mL Needed**

24. meperidine 50 mg
_____

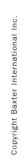

NDC 10019-154-44

Meperidine
HCl Injection, USP

100 mg/mL   R only
FOR INTRAMUSCULAR,
SUBCUTANEOUS OR SLOW
INTRAVENOUS USE
25 x 1 mL DOSETTE® Vials
Baxter   ℮SiLEDERLE®
Mfd. for an affiliate of
Baxter Healthcare Corporation
Deerfield, IL 60015 USA
by: Elkins-Sinn, Inc.
Cherry Hill, NJ 08003
400-854-00

Each mL contains meperidine
HCl 100 mg, sodium metabisul-
fite 1.5 mg and phenol 5 mg in
Water for Injection. Buffered
with acetic acid-sodium acetate.
pH 3.5-6.0. Sealed under nitrogen.

Usual Dosage: See package
insert. Do not use if precipitated.
Store at controlled room temperature 15°-30°C (59°-86°F).

DOSETTE® is a registered trademark
of A.H. Robins Company.

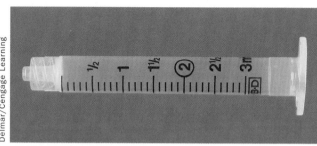

25. clindamycin 0.3 g
_____

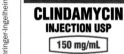

CLINDAMYCIN
INJECTION USP

150 mg/mL

(9 Grams per 60 mL)

PHARMACY BULK PACKAGE
NOT FOR DIRECT INFUSION

FOR INTRAVENOUS USE ONLY
DO NOT DISPENSE AS A UNIT
60 mL PHARMACY BULK PACKAGE
Rx ONLY

NDC 55390-109-01
Usual Dosage: See package insert.

60 mL Pharmacy Bulk Vial

Warning: Dilute before IV use. Swab vial closure with an antiseptic solution. Dispense aliquots
from the vial via a suitable dispensing device into infusion fluids under a laminar flow hood
using aseptic technique. DISCARD VIAL WITHIN 4 HOURS AFTER INITIAL ENTRY.
Store at 20° to 25°C (68° to 77°F); see USP controlled room temperature. Do not refrigerate.
Each mL contains clindamycin phosphate equivalent to clindamycin 150 mg; also disodium
edetate 0.5 mg; benzyl alcohol 9.45 mg added as preservative. When necessary, pH was
adjusted with sodium hydroxide and/or hydrochloric acid.
THIS PHARMACY BULK PACKAGE IS INTENDED FOR PREPARING MANY SINGLE DOSES IN
A PHARMACY ADMIXTURE PROGRAM. FURTHER DILUTION IS REQUIRED. SEE INSERT FOR
FURTHER INFORMATION.

DATE/TIME ENTERED _____   CLND-V00

Manufactured for: Bedford Laboratories™, Bedford, OH 44146

VIAL HANGER LABEL - SLIDE HANGER   OVER VIAL BASE FOR IV ADMINISTRATION

26. morphine sulfate 15 mg
_____

NDC 10019-179-44

Morphine
Sulfate Inj., USP

15 mg/mL
FOR SC, IM OR
SLOW IV USE
1 mL
DOSETTE® Vial
PROTECT FROM LIGHT
DO NOT USE
IF PRECIPITATED
Mfd. for an affiliate of
Baxter Healthcare Corporation
by: Elkins-Sinn
Cherry Hill, NJ 08003
400-833-00

Lot:

Exp.:

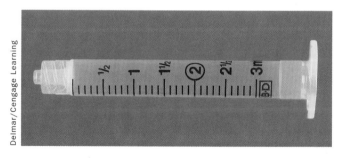

Dosage Ordered	**mL Needed**

27. acyclovir Na 150 mg

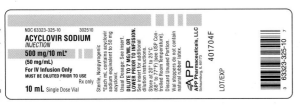

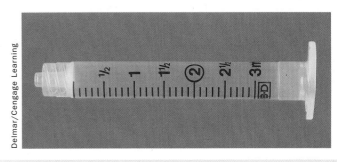

_____

28. cisplatin 20 mg

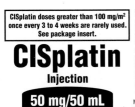

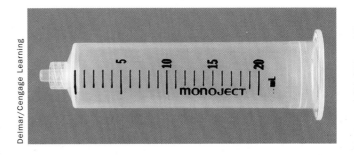

_____

29. sodium chloride 20 mEq

_____

Dosage Ordered

mL Needed

30. meperidine 50 mg

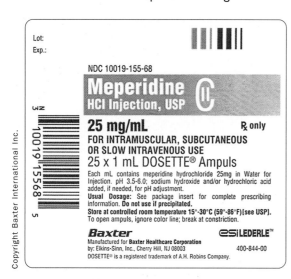

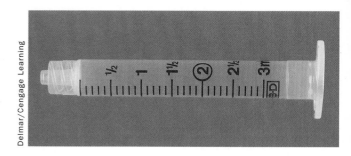

31. furosemide 30 mg

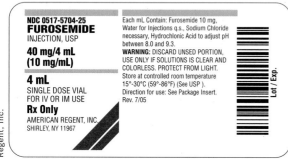

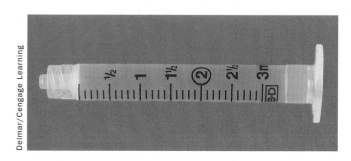

32. gentamicin 60 mg

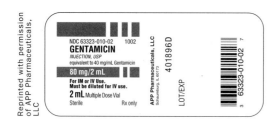

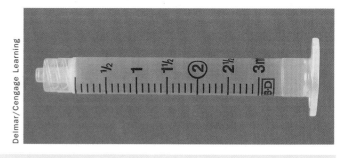

Dosage Ordered   **mL Needed**

33. meperidine 50 mg   _____

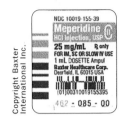

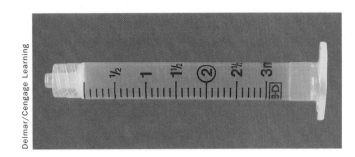

34. dexamethasone 2 mg   _____

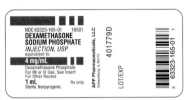

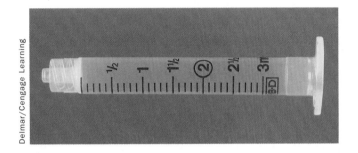

35. Vistaril® 50 mg   _____

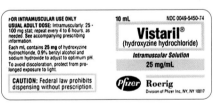

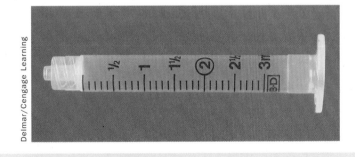

Dosage Ordered	**mL Needed**
36. fentanyl 0.05 mg	

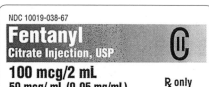

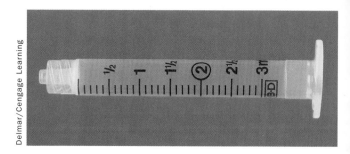

37. morphine 15 mg

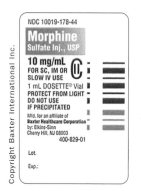

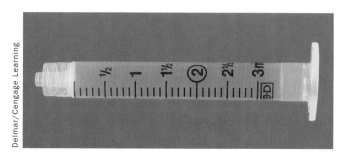

38. cyanocobalamin 1 mg

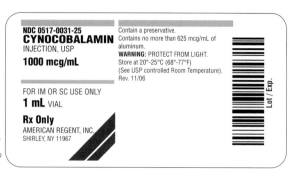

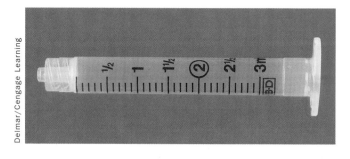

Dosage Ordered   **mL Needed**

39. ketorolac tromethamine 15 mg   _____

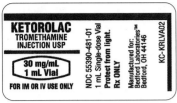

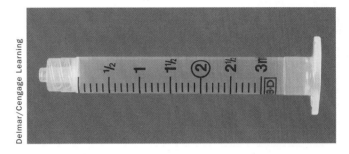

40. Robinul 200 mcg   _____

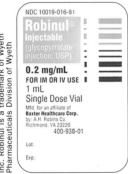

Answers	**9.** 10 mL	**18.** 0.5 mL	**27.** 3 mL	**36.** 1 mL
1. 0.5 mL	**10.** 1 mL	**19.** 2 mL	**28.** 20 mL	**37.** 1.5 mL
2. 1 mL	**11.** 0.5 mL	**20.** 1.5 mL	**29.** 5 mL	**38.** 1 mL
3. 0.5 mL	**12.** 2 mL	**21.** 5 mL	**30.** 2 mL	**39.** 0.5 mL
4. 2 mL	**13.** 2.5 mL	**22.** 10 mL	**31.** 3 mL	**40.** 1 mL
5. 2 mL	**14.** 2 mL	**23.** 2 mL	**32.** 1.5 mL	
6. 1 mL	**15.** 2 mL	**24.** 0.5 mL	**33.** 2 mL	
7. 0.5 mL	**16.** 0.5 mL	**25.** 2 mL	**34.** 0.5 mL	
8. 5 mL	**17.** 1.5 mL	**26.** 1 mL	**35.** 2 mL	

RECONSTITUTION OF POWDERED DRUGS

Objectives

The learner will:

1. prepare solutions from powdered drugs using directions printed on vial labels.

2. prepare solutions from powdered drugs using drug literature or inserts.

3. determine the expiration date and time for reconstituted drugs.

4. calculate dosages for reconstituted drugs.

Many drugs are shipped in powdered form because they **retain their potency only a short time in solution**. Reconstitution of these drugs is often the responsibility of clinical pharmacies, but you will need to know how to read and follow reconstitution directions and how to label drugs with an expiration date and time once they have been reconstituted. The drug label, or instructional package insert, will give specific directions for reconstitution of the drug. Reading these requires care, and this chapter will take you step by step through the entire process.

RECONSTITUTION OF A SINGLE STRENGTH SOLUTION

Let's start with the simplest type of reconstitution instructions, for a single strength solution. Examine the label for the Solu-Medrol® 500 mg vial in Figure 10-1.

Used with permission from Pfizer Inc.

℞ only

81236590 9

See package insert for complete product information. Store at controlled room temperature 20° to 25°C (68° to 77°F) [see USP]. Protect from light. Reconstitute with 8 mL Bacteriostatic Water for Injection with Benzyl Alcohol. **When reconstituted as directed each 8 mL contains:**

*Methylprednisolone sodium succinate equivalent to 500 mg methylprednisolone (62.5 mg per mL). Store solution at controlled room temperature 20° to 25°C (68° to 77°F) [see USP] and use within 48 hours after mixing. Lyophilized in container. Protect from light.

Reconstituted: _____

Pharmacia & Upjohn Co., Kalamazoo, MI 49001, USA

NDC 0009-0758-01
4—125 mg doses

Solu-Medrol®

methylprednisolone sodium succinate for injection, USP

500 mg*

For intramuscular or intravenous use

Diluent Contains Benzyl Alcohol as a Preservative

Figure 10-1

Reconstitution directions on vial labels may be small and difficult to read, and extreme care in reading them is essential.

The first step in reconstitution is to locate the directions. They are on the left side of this label.

Locate the **Reconstitute with 8 mL Bacteriostatic Water for injection with Benzyl Alcohol** instructions. Water, or any other solution specified for reconstitution, is called the **diluent**. The **type of diluent** specified will be **different for different drugs**. The **volume of diluent will also vary**. Therefore, reading the label carefully to identify both the type and the volume of diluent to be used is mandatory.

Once the type of diluent is identified, the next step is to use a **sterile syringe and aseptic technique** to draw up the 8 mL volume required. Inject it slowly into the vial **above the medication level, because air bubbles can distort drug dosages**. If the diluent volume is large, as in this case, be aware that **the syringe plunger will be forced out to expel air to reequalize the internal vial pressure as you inject**. Very large volumes of diluent will have to be injected in divided amounts to keep the internal vial pressure equalized. When all the diluent has been injected, the vial is rotated and upended until all the medication has been dissolved. **Do not shake** unless directed to do so, because this also can add air bubbles to some medications and distort dosages.

After reconstitution locate the information that relates to the **length of time the reconstituted solution may be stored**, and **how it must be stored**. Look again at the Solu-Medrol directions and locate this information. You will find that this solution can be stored at room temperature and that it must be used within 48 hours of reconstitution.

The next step is to **print your initials on the label as the person who reconstituted the drug**, in case any questions subsequently arise concerning the preparation. Next, **add the expiration date and time to the label**. Let's assume you reconstituted this Solu-Medrol solution at **2 pm on January 3**. What expiration (EXP) date and time will you print on the label? The reconstituted drug lasts only 48 hours at room temperature, so you would print **Exp. Jan. 5, 2 pm**, which is 48 hours (2 days) from the time you reconstituted it.

The person who reconstitutes a drug is responsible for labeling it with the date and time of expiration, and with his or her initials.

Next, identify the total dosage strength of this vial, which is **500 mg**. Near the top of the label, you can locate the individual dosage strength: **4–125 mg doses**. Because you have injected 8 mL of diluent, this will be approximately **2 mL for each 125 mg** dose, but if you read the small print on the label, you will see that the individual dosage is clearly identified as **62.5 mg per mL**.

Reconstituted volumes do not always exactly equal the amount of diluent added; in fact, most do not. This is because the medication itself has a volume, and it usually makes the total volume somewhat larger than the amount of diluent injected. Our next examples of a single-strength reconstitution will illustrate this increased volume concept.

If a 62.5 mg dosage is ordered, you will need 1 mL.

If a 125 mg dosage is needed, you will need 2 mL (125 mg = 62.5 mg × 2).

If a 250 mg dosage is needed, you will need 4 mL; and if 500 mg is ordered, the total is 8 mL.

Reconstituted volumes may exceed the volume of the diluent added, because the drug itself has a volume.

Problems 10.1

Other drugs shipped in powdered form are antibiotics. Read the label in Figure 10-2 to answer the following questions about reconstituting this drug. All the information you need is printed sideways on the right of the label.

1. How should this drug be stored before reconstitution? _____

2. How is this drug administered? _____

3. How long will this solution retain its potency at room temperature after reconstitution? _____

4. How long if refrigerated? _____

5. If you reconstitute this drug at 10:10 am on October 3 and it is refrigerated, what expiration time will you print on the label? _____

6. What else will you print on the label? _____

7. What is the total dosage of this reconstituted IV solution? _____

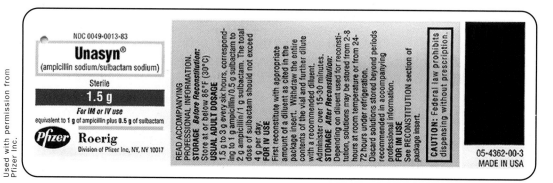

Figure 10-2

Answers 1. at or below 86°F (30°C) **2.** IM or IV **3.** 2–8 hours **4.** 24–72 hours **5.** Exp. Oct. 4 10:10 am to Oct. 6 10:10 am (your answer must include "Exp." to be correct) **6.** Your initials **7.** 1.5 g

---

Problems 10.2

Refer to the penicillin V potassium oral suspension label in Figure 10-3 to answer the following questions.

1. How much diluent is needed to reconstitute this large-volume oral suspension preparation? _____

2. What kind of diluent will you use? _____

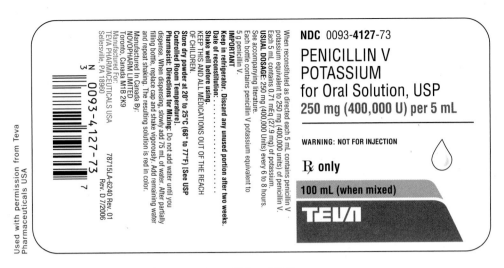

Figure 10-3

3. The label is specific about how to add this diluent. What does it tell you?   _____

4. This is an oral suspension. Does the diluent need to be sterile?   _____

5. What is the mg dosage strength of the prepared solution?   _____

6. Determine the expiration date if you reconstitute this drug on March 15 at 4:40 pm.   _____

7. How must the reconstituted solution be stored?   _____

8. If the dosage ordered is 125 mg, how many mL are needed?   _____

9. For a 500 mg dosage, how many mL are needed?   _____

10. How many units of medication will there be in a 5 mL dose?   _____

11. What should you do to this medication before administering it?   _____

12. What must the person who reconstitutes the medication print on the label?   _____

Answers   1. 75 mL   **2.** Water   **3.** Slowly add water, partially fill bottle and shake vigorously. Add remaning water and shake   **4.** No, this is an oral medication   **5.** 250 mg/5 mL   **6.** Exp. March 29 4:40 pm   **7.** In a refrigerator   **8.** 2.5 mL   **9.** 10 mL   **10.** 400,000 units   **11.** Shake well   **12.** Her initials

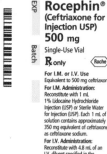

Rocephin®
(Ceftriaxone for
Injection USP)
500 mg
Single-Use Vial

R only   ⟨Roche⟩

For I.M. or I.V. Use
Equivalent to 500 mg ceftriaxone
For I.M. Administration:
Reconstitute with 1 mL
1% Lidocaine Hydrochloride
Injection (USP) or Sterile Water
for Injection (USP). Each 1 mL of
solution contains approximately
350 mg equivalent of ceftriaxone
as ceftriaxone sodium.
For I.V. Administration:
Reconstitute with 4.8 mL of an
I.V. diluent specified in the
accompanying package insert.
Each 1 mL of solution contains
approximately 100 mg equivalent
of ceftriaxone as ceftriaxone
sodium. **Withdraw entire**
contents and dilute to the desired
concentration with the appropriate
I.V. diluent. USUAL DOSAGE: See
package insert.
Storage Prior to Reconstitution:
Store at 20°–25°C (68°–77°F) [see
USP Controlled Room Temperature].
Protect From Light.
Storage After Reconstitution:
See package insert.
Made in Switzerland
Distributed by:
Roche Laboratories Inc.
Nutley, New Jersey 07110

(01) 103 0004 1963 02 7

Figure 10-4

Problems 10.3

Refer to the Rocephin® label in Figure 10-4 to answer the following questions.

1. What is the total dosage of this vial? _____
2. How much diluent is used for IM reconstitution? _____
3. What kind of diluent is specified for IM reconstitution? _____
4. What dosage will 1 mL of IM reconstituted solution contain? _____
5. What is the generic name of this drug? _____
6. How many mL must be added for IV reconstitution? _____
7. Where does it tell you to look for information on the kind of diluent to use for IV reconstitution? _____
8. What dosage will 1 mL of reconstituted IV solution contain? _____
9. Where will you find storage and expiration details? _____
10. What will you print on the label in addition to the expiration date? _____

Answers 1. 500 mg **2.** 1 mL **3.** 1% lidocaine hydrochloride injection or sterile water for injection
4. 350 mg **5.** ceftriaxone **6.** 4.8 mL **7.** Package insert **8.** 100 mg **9.** Package insert **10.** Your initials

Problems 10.4

Refer to the clindamycin label provided in Figure 10-5 to answer the following questions.

1. What is the total dosage in this vial? _____
2. Where will you locate reconstitution instructions? _____
3. How long may the reconstituted solution be used? _____
4. How much clindamycin will a 6 mL IV volume contain? _____
5. How many mL will be needed for a 1500 mg IV dosage? _____
6. What is the mL strength of the reconstituted solution? _____
7. How is this drug administered? _____

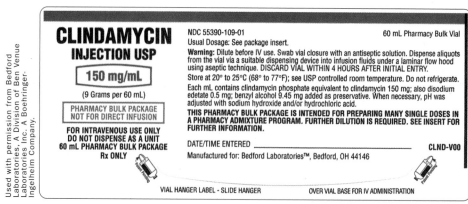

Figure 10-5

Problems 10.5

Refer to the cytarabine label in Figure 10-6 to answer the following questions.

1. What is the total dosage strength of this vial?   _____
2. How much diluent is required for reconstitution?   _____
3. What will be the dosage strength per mL of the
   reconstituted solution?   _____
4. What type of diluent is to be used?   _____
5. How long can the reconstituted solution be retained?   _____
6. How is this medication administered?   _____

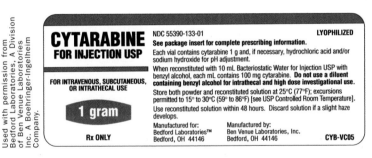

Figure 10-6

Problems 10.6

Refer to the cytarabine label in Figure 10-7 to answer the following questions.

1. What is the total dosage strength of this vial?   _____
2. How much diluent is required for reconstitution?   _____
3. What will be the dosage per mL of the reconstituted
   solution?   _____
4. What is the expiration time of the reconstituted solution?   _____
5. What diluent must be used for subcutaneous injection?   _____

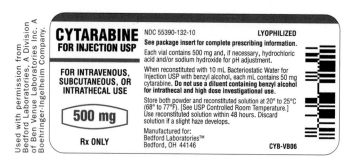

Figure 10-7

Answers **1.** 500 mg **2.** 10 mL **3.** 50 mg per mL **4.** 48 hours **5.** Bacteriostatic water USP with benzyl alcohol

RECONSTITUTION FROM PACKAGE INSERT DIRECTIONS

The package insert directions provided represent just a small portion of the information that drug package inserts contain. Additional information includes specific use of the drug for diagnosed conditions, such as bacterial meningitis, infections of the gastrointestinal or genitourinary tracts, and so forth; dosage recommendations if the vial label does not contain them; and untoward or adverse reactions, to name just a sample of the topics covered.

Problems 10.7

Refer to the selected package insert information in Figure 10-8 to answer the following questions.

1. Identify the types of diluent that may be used for reconstitution under the section labeled **For Intramuscular Use**.   _____

2. Look next at the four-column table for reconstitution, and notice that information is provided for the four different strengths of vials available: 250 mg, 500 mg, 1 g, and 2 g. What volume of diluent is specified for a 250 mg vial?   _____

3. How much diluent is required for a 500 mg vial?   _____

4. How much diluent is required for a 1 g vial?   _____

5. How much diluent is required for a 2 g vial?   _____

6. The mL dosage strength of all four reconstituted solutions is the same. What is it?   _____

7. Refer to the information under **For Direct Intravenous Use**. How much diluent must be added to the 250 mg or 500 mg vials?   _____

8. What stipulation is made for direct IV administration of the 250 mg and 500 mg reconstituted solution?   _____

9. Locate the caution pertaining to rapid IV administration.   _____

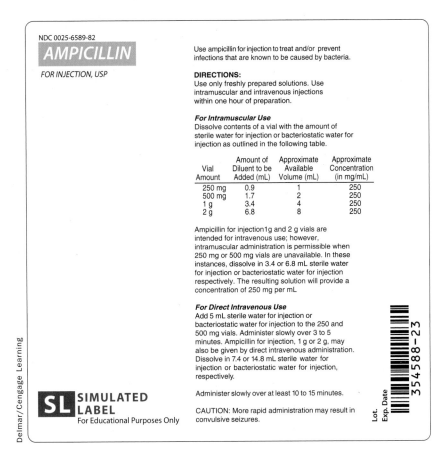

Figure 10-8

Answers **1.** Sterile water for injection or bacteriostatic water for injection   **2.** 0.9 mL   **3.** 1.7 mL
4. 3.4 mL   **5.** 6.8 mL   **6.** 250 mg per 1 mL   **7.** 5 mL   **8.** Inject slowly over 3 to 5 minutes   **9.** Rapid administration may result in seizures

In this section, you were concentrating specifically on locating vial label and package insert directions for reconstitution of a single strength solution. And you quickly discovered that there is no standard way that this information is presented. But the information is all there somewhere; you must persist until you locate it.

The next section will introduce you to labels and package inserts that contain directions for preparation of multiple strength solutions.

RECONSTITUTION OF MULTIPLE STRENGTH SOLUTIONS

Some powdered drugs offer a choice of dosage strengths. When this is the case, you must choose the strength most appropriate for the dosage ordered. For example, refer to the penicillin label in Figure 10-9. The dosage strengths that can be obtained are listed on the right.

SEE ACCOMPANYING PRESCRIBING INFORMATION.	NDC 0049-0530-28	USUAL DOSAGE 6 to 40 million units daily by intravenous infusion only.

Buffered

Pfizerpen®
(penicillin G potassium)

RECOMMENDED STORAGE IN DRY FORM.

Store below 86°F (30°C).

Buffered with sodium citrate and citric acid to optimum pH.

AFTER RECONSTITUTION, SOLUTION SHOULD BE REFRIGERATED. DISCARD UNUSED SOLUTION AFTER 7 DAYS.

Rx only

MADE IN USA

7488

For Injection

TWENTY MILLION UNITS **20**

FOR INTRAVENOUS INFUSION ONLY

Pfizer Roerig
Division of Pfizer Inc, NY, NY 10017

mL diluent added	Approx. units per mL of solution
75 mL	250,000 u/mL
33 mL	500,000 u/mL
11.5 mL	1,000,000 u/mL

PATIENT _____

ROOM _____

DATE/ _____
TIME
BY _____

05-4211-00-8

Figure 10-9

Notice that three dosage strengths are listed: 250,000 units, 500,000 units, and 1,000,000 units/mL. If the dosage ordered is 500,000 units, the most appropriate strength to mix would be 500,000 units/mL. Read across from this strength, and determine how much diluent must be added to obtain it. The answer is 33 mL. If the dosage ordered is 1,000,000 units, what would be the most appropriate strength to prepare, and how much diluent would this require? The answers are 1,000,000 units/mL and 11.5 mL.

A multiple strength solution requires that you add one additional piece of information to the label after reconstitution: the dosage strength just mixed.

Problems 10.8

Refer to the Pfizerpen® label in Figure 10-9 to answer these additional questions.

1. If you add 75 mL of diluent to prepare a solution of penicillin, what dosage strength will you print on the label? _____

2. Does this prepared solution require refrigeration? _____

3. If you reconstitute it on June 1 at 2 pm, what expiration time and date will you print on the label? _____

4. What is the total dosage strength of this vial? _____

5. What else do you print on the label besides the dosage strength just reconstituted? _____

6. Where will you locate information on the diluent to be used? _____

Answers **1.** 250,000 units per mL **2.** Yes **3.** Exp. June 8 2 pm **4.** 20 million units
5. Your initials **6.** Package insert

The next problems consist of two simulated vial labels with solution strengths of 500 mg and 1 g and a package insert that gives the directions for their reconstitution.

Problems 10.9

Refer to the Antibiotic for Intravenous Use labels and insert in Figures 10-10, 10-11, and 10-12. Use both the insert and label information to answer the following questions.

1. How much diluent must be used to reconstitute a 500 mg vial? _____

2. How much diluent will be needed for a 1 g vial? _____

3. What kind of diluent is specified? _____

4. What is the reconstituted dosage per mL of both of these solutions? _____

5. How long can the solution be used if stored in a refrigerator? _____

6. If the drug is reconstituted on May 4 at 1350, what expiration date and time will you print on the label? _____

7. What else must you print on the label? _____

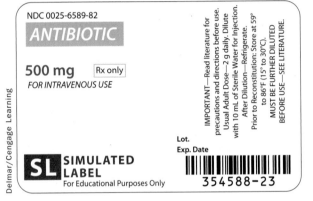

Figure 10-10

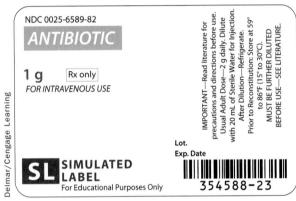

Figure 10-11

> **PREPARATION AND STABILITY**
> At the time of use, reconstitute by adding either 10 mL of Sterile Water for Injection to the 500-mg vial or 20 mL of Sterile Water for Injection to the 1-g vial of dry, sterile powder. Vials reconstituted in this manner will give a solution of 50 mg/mL. FURTHER DILUTION IS REQUIRED.
> After reconsitution, the vials may be stored in a refrigerator for 14 days without significant loss of potency. Reconstituted solutions containing 500 mg must be diluted with at least 100 mL of diluent. Reconstituted solutions containing 1g must be diluted with at least 200 mL of diluent, The desired dose, diluted in this manner, should be administered by intermittent intravenous infusion over a period of at least 60 minutes.

Figure 10-12

Answers   1. 10 mL   **2.** 20 mL   **3.** Sterile water for injection   **4.** 50 mg per mL   **5.** 14 days
6. Exp. May 18 1350   **7.** Your initials

Summary

This concludes the chapter on the reconstitution of powdered drugs. The important points to remember from this chapter are:

▪ If the medication label does not contain reconstitution directions, these may be located on the medication package insert.

📭 The type and amount of diluent to be used for reconstitution must be exactly as specified in the reconstitution instructions.

📭 If directions are given for both IM and IV reconstitution, be careful to read the correct set for the solution you are preparing.

📭 The person who reconstitutes a drug must initial the vial and print the expiration time and date on the label, unless all the drug is used immediately.

📭 If a solution is prepared using multiple strength medication directions, the strength reconstituted must also be printed on the label.

Summary Self-Test

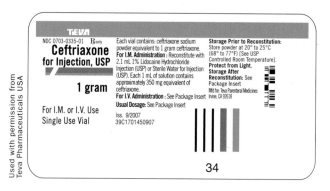

Figure 10-13

Refer to the ceftriaxone label in Figure 10-13 to answer the following questions about reconstitution.

1. What is the total dosage of this vial? _____

2. What volume of diluent must be used for reconstitution? _____

3. What will be the dosage strength of 1 mL of reconstituted solution? _____

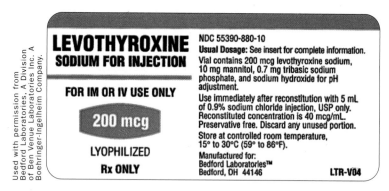

Figure 10-14

Refer to the levothyroxine sodium label in Figure 10-14 to answer the following questions.

4. What is the dosage strength of this vial in mcg? In mg? _____ _____

5. What volume of diluent must you add to prepare the solution for use? _____

6. What kind of diluent must be used? _____

7. How long will this reconstituted solution retain its potency?   _____

8. What is the per mL strength of the reconstituted solution?   _____

9. Where will you find average dosage instructions?   _____

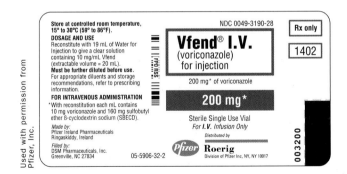

Figure 10-15

Refer to the cytarabine label in Figure 10-15 to answer the following questions.

10. How much diluent is used to reconstitute this solution?   _____

11. What type of diluent?   _____

12. What is the total vial dosage?   _____

13. At what temperature should this medication be stored?   _____

14. What dosage will each 1 mL contain?   _____

15. What is the expiration time of the reconstituted solution?   _____

16. If the solution is reconstituted on Feb 14 at 0840, what expiration
date must be printed on the label?   _____

Figure 10-16

Refer to the VFend® I.V. label in Figure 10-16 to answer the following questions.

17. How much diluent is required to reconstitute this Vfend I.V. solution?   _____

18. What diluent is specified for use?   _____

19. What is the strength of each 1 mL of the reconstituted solution?   _____

20. What is the total dosage of this vial?   _____

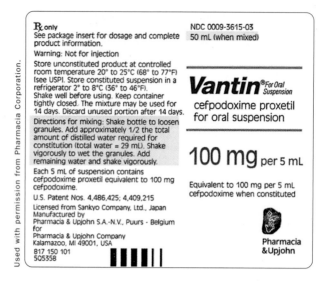

Figure 10-17

Refer to the Vantin® Oral Suspension label in Figure 10-17 to answer the following questions.

21. How much diluent will be required to reconstitute this medication? _____

22. What type of diluent is listed for reconstitution? _____

23. How is this diluent to be added? _____

24. What is the reconstituted dosage strength? _____

25. How long will the reconstituted Vantin solution retain its potency? _____

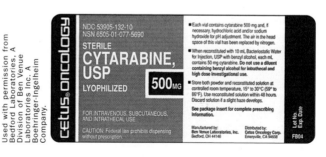

Figure 10-18

Refer to the cytarabine label in Figure 10-18 to answer the following questions.

26. What is the total strength of this medication? _____

27. What diluent must be used for reconstitution? _____

28. How much? _____

29. What is the dosage per reconstituted mL? _____

30. How long does the reconstituted cytarabine solution retain its potency at room temperature? _____

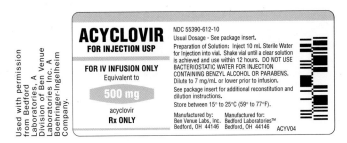

Figure 10-19

Refer to the acyclovir label in Figure 10-19 to answer the following questions for reconstitution.

31. What type of diluent is recommended for reconstitution? _____

32. How much diluent must be added? _____

33. What is the total dosage strength of this vial? _____

34. How soon must this solution be used? _____

Figure 10-20

Refer to the cytarabine label in Figure 10-20 and answer the following questions.

35. What is the total dosage strength of this vial? _____

36. What volume of diluent must be added? _____

37. What kind of diluent must be used? _____

38. What is the reconstituted dosage strength per mL? _____

39. How long will this medication retain its potency? _____

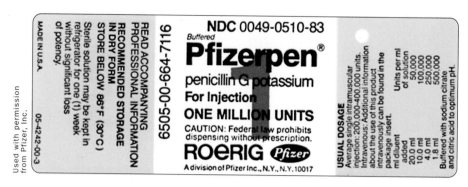

Figure 10-21

Refer to the penicillin G potassium label in Figure 10-21 to answer the following questions.

40. What is the total dosage strength of this vial? _____

41. How much diluent must be added to prepare a 100,000 units/mL strength? _____

42. How much diluent must be added to prepare a 500,000 units/mL strength? _____

43. How much diluent must be added to prepare a 50,000 units/mL strength? _____

44. This label has no information on the type of diluent to use. Where will you find this? _____

45. How must this solution be stored? _____

46. If reconstituted at 1:10 am on December 18, what must you print on the label? _____

47. What else must you print on the label? _____

48. Why print? _____

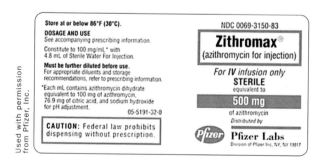

Figure 10-22

Refer to the Zithromax® label in Figure 10-22 to answer the following questions.

49. What is the generic name for Zithromax? _____

50. What is the dosage strength of this vial? _____

51. What diluent is specified for reconstitution? _____

52. How much diluent is required? _____

53. What is the reconstituted dosage strength? _____

Answer

1. 1 g
2. 2.1 mL
3. 350 mg/mL
4. 200 mcg; 0.2 mg
5. 5 mL
6. 0.9% sodium chloride
7. must be used immediately
8. 40 mcg/mL
9. package insert
10. 10 mL
11. Bacteriostatic Water for Injection with Benzyl Alcohol
12. 1 gram
13. 25°C (77°F)
14. 100 mg per mL
15. 48 hours
16. Exp. Feb. 16 0840
17. 19 mL
18. Water for Injection
19. 10 mg/mL
20. 200 mg
21. 29 mL
22. Distilled Water
23. Shake the bottle to loosen granules, add half (15 mL) of the distilled water, and shake vigorously to dissolve granules; add balance of water and shake vigorously
24. 100 mg/5 mL
25. 14 days
26. 500 mg
27. Bacteriostatic Water with Benzyl Alcohol
28. 10 mL
29. 50 mg per mL
30. 48 hours
31. Sterile Water for Injection
32. 10 mL
33. 500 mg
34. Within 12 hours
35. 2 g
36. 20 mL
37. Bacteriostatic Water for Injection USP with Benzyl Alcohol
38. 100 mg/mL
39. 48 hours
40. One million units
41. 10 mL
42. 1.8 mL
43. 20 mL
44. Package insert
45. Refrigerate
46. Exp. 1:10 am Dec. 25
47. Your initials
48. Space considerations; handwriting is difficult to read
49. azithromycin
50. 500 mg
51. Sterile Water for Injection
52. 4.8 mL
53. 100 mg per mL

4

Dosage Calculations

12

DIMENSIONAL ANALYSIS/UNITS CONVERSION

Objectives

The learner will:

1. use dimensional analysis to calculate dosages.

Prerequisites

Chapters 1–10

You may already be familiar with dimensional analysis (DA) under its official name: **units conversion**, which is used in chemistry, physics, and other scientific calculations. DA was first introduced for clinical dosage calculations in the 1950s using the name dimensional analysis, but it has acquired several other names along the way: the label factor and factor label methods being two.

DA is actually ratio and proportion made simple. Its great virtue is that **it reduces multiple-step calculations to a single equation**. However, to understand the simplicity of DA, it is necessary to look at clinical ratios from a different perspective.

CLINICAL RATIOS

Clinical ratios provide the components for **all** the calculations you have already learned and will be learning in the remainder of this text. Some examples of ratios you are already familiar with from previous chapters include the following:

> **oral dosages:** 1 tab = 250 mg; 5 mL = 125 mg
> **IM and subcutaneous dosages:** 2 g = 1.5 mL;
> 1 mL = 10 units; 10 mL = 20 mEq
> **metric conversions:** 1000 mcg = 1 mg; 1 g = 1000 mg

In addition, you will be using the following ratios, although it isn't necessary for you to memorize them at this time.

> **IV flow rates:** 80 gtt per min; 100 mL per hr
> **IV set calibrations:** 10 gtt per mL; 15 gtt per mL; 60 gtt per mL
> **time conversions:** 60 min = 1 hr; 1 hr = 60 min

In DA, ratios are written as common fractions.

$$\frac{1 \text{ tab}}{250 \text{ mg}} \qquad \frac{5 \text{ mL}}{125 \text{ mg}} \qquad \frac{2 \text{ g}}{1.5 \text{ mL}}$$

$$\frac{1 \text{ mL}}{10 \text{ units}} \qquad \frac{10 \text{ mL}}{20 \text{ mEq}} \qquad \frac{1000 \text{ mcg}}{1 \text{ mg}}$$

THE BASIC DA EQUATION

The first step in setting up a DA equation is to **write the unit of measure being calculated**. One commonly calculated measure is mL, so let's begin by using an mL calculation to illustrate the steps involved. Notice that color is used in the first DA examples to help you learn the sequence of ratio entry.

EXAMPLE 1   The available dosage strength is **750 mg in 2.5 mL**. How many mL will be needed to prepare a **600 mg** dosage?

Write the mL unit of measure being calculated, followed by an equal sign.

$$mL \; =$$

There are two important reasons for identifying the unit of measure being calculated first: it eliminates any confusion over exactly **which** measure is being calculated, and it dictates how the first or "starting" clinical ratio is entered in the equation.

In a DA equation, the unit of measure being calculated is written first, followed by an equal sign.

Next, go back to the problem to **identify the complete clinical ratio that contains mL**. This is provided by the **dosage strength available**, which is **750 mg in 2.5 mL**. Enter this as a common fraction so that **the 2.5 mL *numerator* matches the mL unit of measure being calculated; 750 mg** becomes **the *denominator***.

$$mL \; = \; \frac{2.5 \; mL}{750 \; mg}$$

In a DA equation, the unit of measure being calculated is matched in the numerator of the first clinical ratio entered.

All additional ratios are entered so that **each *denominator* is matched in its successive *numerator***. The **denominator in the first ratio is mg**, so the **next numerator must be mg**. Go back to the problem to discover that this is provided by the **600 mg** dosage to be given. Enter this now as the next numerator to complete this single-step equation.

$$mL \; = \; \frac{2.5 \; mL}{750 \; mg} \times \frac{600 \; mg}{}$$

The unit of measure in each denominator of a DA equation is matched in the successive numerator entered.

All the pertinent clinical ratios have now been entered in this one-step DA equation. The next step is to **cancel the alternate denominator/numerator measurement units (but not their quantities) to be sure they match**. This ensures that the clinical ratios were entered correctly. **After cancellation, only the unit of measure being calculated may remain in the equation**. The denominator/numerator mg/mg units cancel, leaving only the mL unit being calculated remaining in the equation.

$$mL \; = \; \frac{2.5 \; mL}{750 \; \cancel{mg}} \times \frac{600 \; \cancel{mg}}{}$$

Only the unit of measure being calculated may remain in the equation after the denominator/numerator units of measure are cancelled.

Only the mL being calculated remains in the equation. The math can now be done.

$$mL = \frac{2.5 \text{ mL}}{750 \text{ mg}} \times \frac{600 \text{ mg}}{}$$

$$mL = \frac{2.5 \text{ mL}}{\underset{5}{750} \text{ mg}} \times \frac{\overset{4}{600} \text{ mg}}{} \qquad \text{Divide by 150}$$

$$mL = \frac{\overset{2}{10}}{\underset{1}{5}} = 2 \text{ mL}$$

To obtain a dosage of 600 mg from an available dosage strength of 750 mg in 2.5 mL, you would give 2 mL.

DA works exactly the same way for every calculation **regardless of the number of ratios entered**. As you can see, there are no complicated rules to memorize. In these simple steps, you have now learned how to use DA for **all** clinical calculations.

EXAMPLE 2 A dosage of **50,000 units** is ordered to be added to an IV solution. The strength available is **10,000 units in 1.5 mL**. Calculate how many **mL** will contain this dosage.

Write the mL being calculated to the left of the equation followed by an equal sign.

$$mL =$$

Locate the complete ratio containing mL, the 10,000 units in 1.5 mL dosage strength available. Enter this now, with **1.5 mL as the numerator to match the mL being calculated**; 10,000 units becomes the denominator.

$$mL = \frac{1.5 \text{ mL}}{10,000 \text{ units}}$$

The units denominator must be matched in the next numerator. This is provided by the 50,000 units ordered. Enter this now to complete this one-step equation.

$$mL = \frac{1.5 \text{ mL}}{10,000 \text{ units}} \times \frac{50,000 \text{ units}}{}$$

Cancel the alternate denominator/numerator units/units entries to double-check for correct ratio entry. Only the mL being calculated remains in the equation. Do the math.

$$mL = \frac{1.5 \text{ mL}}{10,000 \text{ units}} \times \frac{50,000 \text{ units}}{}$$

$$mL = \frac{1.5 \text{ mL}}{10,000 \text{ units}} \times \frac{\overset{5}{50,000} \text{ units}}{1} \qquad \begin{array}{l}\text{Divide 50,000 by 10,000 to}\\ \text{obtain 5; multiply 1.5 by 5 to}\\ \text{obtain 7.5 mL}\end{array}$$

$$mL = 1.5 \times 5 = 7.5 \text{ mL}$$

It will require a 7.5 mL volume of the 10,000 units in 1.5 mL solution to prepare the 50,000 units ordered for this IV additive.

EXAMPLE 3   Tablet calculations are not common but would be done the same way using DA.

Scored (breakable) **tablets** with a strength of **0.5 mg** are available to prepare a dosage of **1.25 mg**. How many **tablets** must you give?

Enter the tab being calculated to the left of the equation followed by an equal sign.

$$\text{tab} =$$

The tab unit being calculated is matched by the tab strength available, 0.5 mg in 1 tab. Enter this as the first ratio, with 1 tab as the numerator; 0.5 mg becomes the denominator.

$$\text{tab} = \frac{1 \text{ tab}}{0.5 \text{ mg}}$$

The mg denominator must be matched in the next numerator. This is provided by the 1.25 mg ordered. Enter this to complete the equation.

$$\text{tab} = \frac{1 \text{ tab}}{0.5 \text{ mg}} \times \frac{1.25 \text{ mg}}{}$$

Cancel the alternate denominator/numerator mg units of measure to check that you have entered the ratios correctly. Only the tab being calculated remains in the equation. Do the math.

$$\text{tab} = \frac{1 \text{ tab}}{0.5 \text{ \cancel{mg}}} \times \frac{1.25 \text{ \cancel{mg}}}{}$$

$$\text{tab} = \frac{1 \text{ tab}}{\cancel{50} \text{ \cancel{mg}}_2} \times \frac{\cancel{125}^{5} \text{ \cancel{mg}}}{}$$ Eliminate the decimal points; reduce the numbers

$$\text{tab} = \frac{5}{2} = 2\frac{1}{2} \text{ tab}$$

To obtain the 1.25 mg dosage ordered, 2½ tab must be given.

Let's stop for a moment now and take a look at what happens if the ratios are incorrectly entered in a DA equation. We'll **assume that the units of measure have not been entered with their quantities** and that the **entries have been mixed up**. The correct equation will be shown alongside for comparison.

EXAMPLE 4   A drug label reads **100 mg per 2 mL**. The medication order is for **130 mg**. How many **mL** must you prepare?

Correct   **Incorrect**

$$\text{mL} = \frac{2 \text{ mL}}{100 \text{ mg}} \times \frac{130 \text{ mg}}{} = 2.6 \text{ mL} \qquad \text{mL} = \frac{100}{2} \times \frac{130}{} = 6500 \text{ mL}$$

In the incorrect equation, the starting ratio is upside down, and since the units of measure were not entered with their quantities, there is no way to catch this.

The safety step of cancellation to check ratio entry cannot be done. But notice something else: The answer, 6500 mL, is impossible. If the entries in a DA equation are mixed up, the numbers are often so outrageous that you will know instantly that you have made a mistake. **But mistakes are not always this obvious, so stick to the step-by-step calculation rules**. There is a reason for every one of them. Let's look at a few more examples.

EXAMPLE 5 How many **mL** will you draw up to prepare a **1.2 g** dosage if the solution available is labeled **2 g in 3 mL**?

Write the mL unit being calculated to the left of the equation followed by an equal sign. Enter the starting ratio, 2 g in 3 mL, with 3 mL as the numerator to match the mL being calculated; 2 g becomes the denominator.

$$mL = \frac{3\ mL}{2\ g}$$

Match the g denominator in the next numerator with the 1.2 g ordered to complete the equation.

$$mL = \frac{3\ mL}{2\ g} \times \frac{1.2\ g}{}$$

Cancel the alternate denominator/numerator g units of measure to double-check that the entries are correct. Only the mL being calculated remains.

$$mL = \frac{3\ mL}{2\ \cancel{g}} \times \frac{1.2\ \cancel{g}}{}$$

Do the math, expressing fractional answers to the nearest tenth.

$$mL = \frac{3\ mL}{2\ \cancel{g}} \times \frac{1.2\ \cancel{g}}{} = \textbf{1.8 mL}$$

The 1.2 g dosage ordered is contained in 1.8 mL of the 2 g in 3 mL solution available.

EXAMPLE 6 Medication with a strength of **0.75 mg per mL** is available to prepare a dosage of **2 mg**. Calculate the mL this will require.

Write the mL being calculated to the left of the equation followed by an equal sign.

$$mL =$$

The mL being calculated is provided for the first ratio by the 0.75 mg per mL dosage strength available. Enter 1 mL as the numerator and 0.75 mg as the denominator.

$$mL = \frac{1\ mL}{0.75\ mg}$$

The mg denominator must now be matched. This is provided by the 2 mg dosage ordered. Enter this now to complete this one-step equation.

$$mL = \frac{1\ mL}{0.75\ mg} \times \frac{2\ mg}{}$$

Cancel the alternate denominator/numerator mg units of measure to check for correct ratio entry, then do the math.

$$mL = \frac{1 \text{ mL}}{0.75 \text{ mg}} \times \frac{2 \text{ mg}}{} = 2.67 = \textbf{2.7 mL}$$

It will require 2.7 mL of the 0.75 mg in 1 mL dosage available to administer the 2 mg ordered.

Problems 12.1

Calculate these dosages using DA. Express mL answers to the nearest tenth.

1. A dosage of 0.3 g has been ordered. The strength available is 0.4 g in 1.5 mL.   _____

2. A dosage strength of 0.8 mg in 2 mL is to be used to prepare a 0.5 mg dosage.   _____

3. Prepare a 1.8 mg dosage from a solution labeled 2 mg in 3 mL.   _____

4. The order is for 1500 mg. You have available a 1200 mg per mL solution.   _____

5. A dosage strength of 0.2 mg in 1.5 mL is available. Give 0.15 mg.   _____

6. The strength available is 1000 mg in 3.6 mL. Prepare a 600 mg dosage.   _____

7. A 10,000 units dosage has been ordered. The strength available is 8000 units in 1 mL.   _____

8. An IV additive has a dosage strength of 20 mEq per 20 mL. A dosage of 15 mEq has been ordered.   _____

9. A 200,000 units dosage must be prepared from a 150,000 units in 2 mL strength.   _____

10. An IV additive order is for 400 mg. The solution available has a strength of 500 mg in 20 mL.   _____

Answers   1. 1.1 mL   **2.** 1.3 mL   **3.** 2.7 mL   **4.** 1.3 mL   **5.** 1.1 mL   **6.** 2.2 mL   **7.** 1.3 mL   **8.** 15 mL
9. 2.7 mL   **10.** 16 mL

You now know the basics of using DA in calculations. **But how do you know if the answer you obtain is correct?** The answer to this question is provided by the key points already covered.

- **If** the unit being calculated is correctly identified to the left of the equation.
- **If** the starting ratio is entered so that its numerator matches the unit of measure being calculated.
- **If** the unit of measure in each denominator is matched in each successively entered numerator.

- **If** the only unit of measure remaining after cancellation is the same as the unit of measure being calculated.
- **If** the quantities have been correctly entered.
- **If** the math has been double-checked and is correct.

THEN THE ANSWER WILL BE CORRECT.

A tall order? Not really. You are doing a clinical dosage calculation. All you must do is carefully follow each step, and the answer will be correct.

In addition, **don't divorce your previous learning and reasoning from the calculation process.** You already know that **most IM dosages are contained in a 0.5–3 mL volume,** that **IV additives may be contained in larger volumes,** and that **large numbers of tab/cap are unusual** in dosages. **If you get an unreasonable answer to a calculation, you must question it.** In time, you will know the average dosages of all the drugs you give and another safety component will be added to your repertoire, but for now, concentrate on the simple mechanics of calculation you have just been taught. Don't shortcut these steps, and you'll do just fine.

EQUATIONS REQUIRING METRIC CONVERSIONS

The major advantage of DA is that it allows multiple ratios to be entered in a single equation. This is especially useful when a drug is ordered in one unit of measure—for example, mg—but is labeled in another—for example, g or mcg.

There are two ways to handle a conversion. Sometimes, it will be easier to do the conversion before setting up the equation. In other instances, you may elect to incorporate the conversion into an equation. For practice purposes, let's look at how **conversion ratios**—for example, **1 g = 1000 mg** or **1 mg = 1000 mcg**—are entered in a DA equation.

EXAMPLE 1   The IM dosage ordered is **275 mg**. The drug available is labeled **0.5 g per 2 mL**. How many **mL** must you give?

Enter the mL to be calculated to the left of the equation. Locate the ratio containing mL, the 0.5 g per 2 mL dosage strength, and enter it, with 2 mL as the numerator; 0.5 g becomes the denominator.

$$\text{mL} = \frac{2\,\text{mL}}{0.5\,\text{g}}$$

When you refer back to the problem, you will not find a g measure to match the starting ratio g denominator. The dosage to be given is in mg. So, a **conversion ratio between g and mg** is needed: 1 g = 1000 mg. Enter this now, with **1 g as the numerator to match the g of the previous denominator**; 1000 mg becomes the new denominator.

$$\text{mL} = \frac{2\,\text{mL}}{0.5\,\text{g}} \times \frac{1\,\text{g}}{1000\,\text{mg}}$$

The final entry, the 275 mg dosage to be given, will automatically fall into its correct position as it is entered as the final numerator to match the mg of the previous denominator. The equation is now complete.

$$mL = \frac{2\ mL}{0.5\ g} \times \frac{1\ g}{1000\ mg} \times \frac{275\ mg}{}$$

Cancel the alternate denominator/numerator g/g and mg/mg units of measure to double-check the ratio entry. Only the mL being calculated remains. Do the math.

$$mL = \frac{2\ mL}{0.5\ \cancel{g}} \times \frac{1\ \cancel{g}}{1000\ \cancel{mg}} \times \frac{275\ \cancel{mg}}{} = \textbf{1.1 mL}$$

To give a dosage of 275 mg, you must prepare 1.1 mL of the 0.5 g in 2 mL strength solution.

EXAMPLE 2   The drug label reads **800 mcg in 1.5 mL**. The IM order is for **0.6 mg**.

Enter the mL to be calculated followed by an equal sign to the left of the equation. Locate the ratio containing mL, 800 mcg in 1.5 mL. Enter 1.5 mL as the numerator to match the mL being calculated; 800 mcg becomes the denominator.

$$mL = \frac{1.5\ mL}{800\ mcg}$$

There is no mcg measure in the problem, which is your clue to the necessity for a conversion ratio. Enter the 1000 mcg = 1 mg conversion ratio, with 1000 mcg as the numerator to match the mcg of the previous denominator; 1 mg becomes the denominator.

$$mL = \frac{1.5\ mL}{800\ mcg} \times \frac{1000\ mcg}{1\ mg}$$

The mg denominator is now matched by the 0.6 mg dosage to be given, and completes the equation.

$$mL = \frac{1.5\ mL}{800\ mcg} \times \frac{1000\ mcg}{1\ mg} \times \frac{0.6\ mg}{}$$

Cancel the alternate denominator/numerator mcg/mcg and mg/mg units of measure to check for correct ratio entry. Only the mL being calculated should remain in the equation. Do the math.

$$mL = \frac{1.5\ mL}{800\ \cancel{mcg}} \times \frac{1000\ \cancel{mcg}}{1\ \cancel{mg}} \times \frac{0.6\ \cancel{mg}}{} = 1.12 = \textbf{1.1 mL}$$

To give a dosage of 0.6 mg from the available 1.5 mL per 800 mcg strength, you must prepare 1.1 mL.

EXAMPLE 3   Prepare a **0.5 mg** dosage from an available strength of **200 mcg per mL**.

Enter the mL being calculated to the left of the equation followed by an equal sign. Enter the 1 mL in 200 mcg dosage as the starting ratio, with 1 mL as the numerator to match the mL being calculated; 200 mcg becomes the denominator.

$$mL = \frac{1 \text{ mL}}{200 \text{ mcg}}$$

A mcg to mg conversion ratio is needed. Enter 1000 mcg as the numerator to match the mcg in the previous denominator; 1 mg becomes the new denominator.

$$mL = \frac{1 \text{ mL}}{200 \text{ mcg}} \times \frac{1000 \text{ mcg}}{1 \text{ mg}}$$

The mg denominator is now matched by the 0.5 mg dosage ordered to complete the equation.

$$mL = \frac{1 \text{ mL}}{200 \text{ mcg}} \times \frac{1000 \text{ mcg}}{1 \text{ mg}} \times \frac{0.5 \text{ mg}}{}$$

Cancel the alternate mcg/mcg and mg/mg units of measure to double-check for correct ratio entry. Only the mL unit being calculated remains in the equation. Do the math.

$$mL = \frac{1 \text{ mL}}{200 \text{ mcg}} \times \frac{1000 \text{ mcg}}{1 \text{ mg}} \times \frac{0.5 \text{ mg}}{} = \textbf{2.5 mL}$$

A 0.5 mg dosage requires a 2.5 mL volume of the 200 mcg per mL strength solution available.

EXAMPLE 4   The medication has a strength of **0.5 g in 1.5 mL**. Prepare **750 mg**.

Enter the mL to be calculated to the left of the equation followed by an equal sign. Enter the starting ratio, the 1.5 mL in 0.5 g dosage available, with 1.5 mL as the numerator, to match the mL being calculated; 0.5 g becomes the denominator.

$$mL = \frac{1.5 \text{ mL}}{0.5 \text{ g}}$$

There is no g dosage in the problem, which signals the need for a conversion ratio. Enter the 1 g = 1000 mg conversion ratio, with 1 g as the numerator, to match the g denominator of the starting ratio; 1000 mg becomes the new denominator.

$$mL = \frac{1.5 \text{ mL}}{0.5 \text{ g}} \times \frac{1 \text{ g}}{1000 \text{ mg}}$$

Enter the dosage ordered, 750 mg, as the final numerator to match the mg in the previous denominator. The equation is complete.

$$mL = \frac{1.5 \text{ mL}}{0.5 \text{ g}} \times \frac{1 \text{ g}}{1000 \text{ mg}} \times \frac{750 \text{ mg}}{}$$

Cancel the alternate g/g and mg/mg units of measure to check the accuracy of ratio entry, then complete the math.

$$mL = \frac{1.5 \text{ mL}}{0.5 \text{ g}} \times \frac{1 \text{ g}}{1000 \text{ mg}} \times \frac{750 \text{ mg}}{} = 2.25 = \textbf{2.3 mL}$$

A 750 mg dosage requires 2.3 mL of the 0.5 g in 1.5 mL medication.

Problems 12.2

Calculate these dosages using DA. Express mL answers to the nearest tenth.

1. Prepare 0.1 g of an IM medication from a strength of
   200 mg per mL.   _____

2. A drug label reads 0.1 g in 2 mL. Prepare a 130 mg dosage. _____

3. An oral solution has a strength of 500 mg in 5 mL. Prepare
   a 0.6 g dosage.   _____

4. Prepare a 0.75 g dosage from a 250 mg per mL strength solution. _____

5. Prepare 500 mg for IM injection from an available strength of
   1 g per 3 mL.   _____

6. A dosage of 85 mg is ordered, and the drug available is labeled
   0.1 g in 1.5 mL.   _____

7. The strength available is 500 mcg in 1.5 mL. Prepare
   a 0.75 mg dosage.   _____

8. A dosage of 1500 mg has been ordered. The solution available
   is 0.5 g per mL.   _____

9. The dosage strength available is 200 mcg per mL. A 0.5 mg
   dosage has been ordered.   _____

10. The dosage ordered is 0.2 g. Tablets available are labeled 80 mg. _____

Answers   1. 0.5 mL   **2.** 2.6 mL   **3.** 6 mL   **4.** 3 mL   **5.** 1.5 mL   **6.** 1.3 mL   **7.** 2.3 mL   **8.** 3 mL
9. 2.5 mL   **10.** 2½ tab

Summary

**This completes your introduction to clinical calculations using dimensional analysis.
The important points to remember from this chapter are:**

- The unit of measure being calculated is written first to the left of the equation, followed by an equal sign.

- All ratios entered must include the quantity **and** the unit of measure.

- The numerator in the starting ratio must be in the same measurement unit as the unit of measure being calculated.

- The unit of measure in each denominator must be matched in the numerator of each successive ratio entered.

- Metric system conversions can be made by incorporating a conversion ratio directly into the DA equation.

- The unit of measure in each alternate denominator and numerator must cancel, leaving only the unit of measure being calculated remaining in the equation.

- The numerator of the starting ratio is never cancelled.

Summary Self-Test

Calculate these dosages using DA. Express mL answers to the nearest tenth (or hundredth where indicated) using the medication labels provided. Measure the dosages you calculate on the syringes provided. Have your answers checked by your instructor to be sure you have calculated and measured the dosages correctly.

Dosage Ordered   **mL Needed**

1. terbutaline sulfate 800 mcg

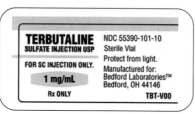
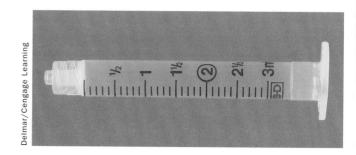

2. furosemide 15 mg

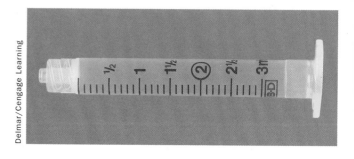

3. Vistaril® 70mg

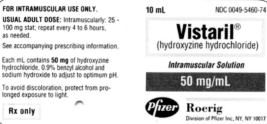
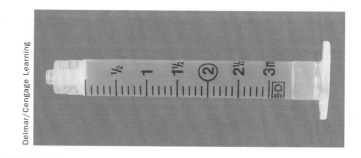

Dosage Ordered   **mL Needed**

4. fentanyl citrate 0.15 mg   _____

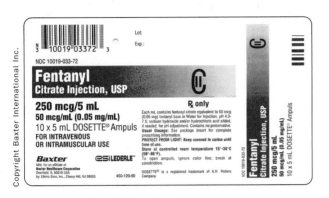

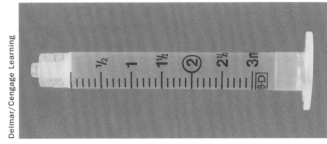

5. naloxone 350 mcg   _____

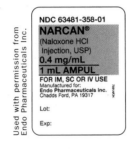

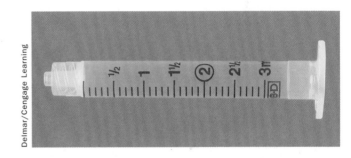

6. clindamycin 225 mg   _____

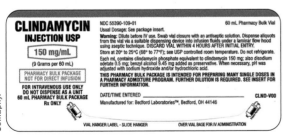

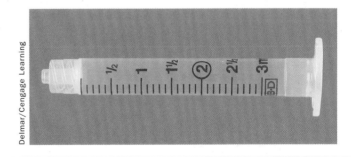

7. Robinul® 75 mcg (calculate to the nearest hundredth)   _____

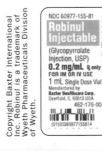

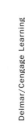

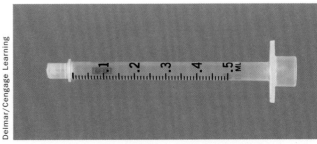

Dosage Ordered	**mL Needed**

8. midazolam HCl 4 mg _____

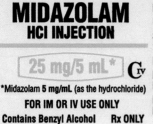

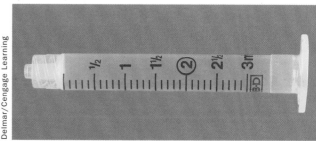

9. Inapsine® 3mg _____

10. cyanocobalamin 800 mcg _____

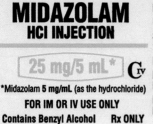

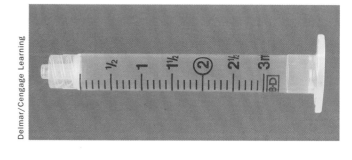

Dosage Ordered   mL Needed

11. potassium acetate 16 mEq for IV additive   _____

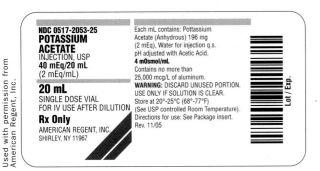

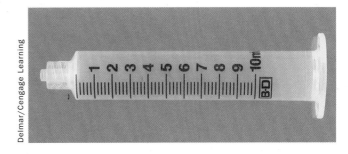

12. calcium gluconate 0.93 mEq for an IV additive   _____

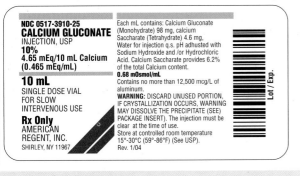

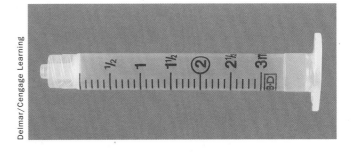

13. morphine sulfate 1.5 mg   _____

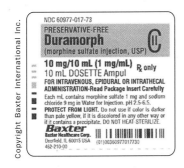

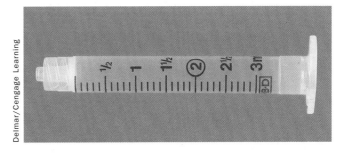

14. heparin sodium 450 units (calculate to the nearest hundredth)   _____

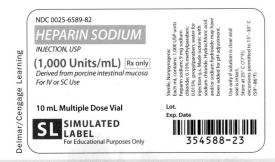

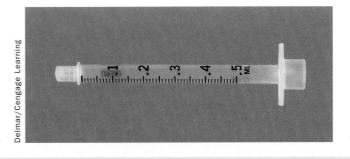

Dosage Ordered   **mL Needed**

15. droperidol 4 mg

_____

NDC 11098-010-02   2 mL ampoule

INAPSINE®

(DROPERIDOL) INJECTION

5 mg/2 mL (2.5 mg/mL)

TAYLOR PHARMACEUTICALS
Decatur, IL 62522

ADPADL   Rev. 3/00

LOT

EXP.

Used with permission from Akorn Inc. and Taylor Pharmaceuticals.

16. Dilantin® 0.1 g

_____

Dosage—See package insert.
℞ only

Manufactured by:
Parkedale Pharmaceuticals, Inc.
Rochester, MI 48307

For:
PARKE-DAVIS
Div of Warner-Lambert Co
Morris Plains, NJ 07950 USA

N 0071-4475-45
STERI-VIAL®
Dilantin®
(Phenytoin Sodium Injection, USP)
ready/mixed

250 mg in 5 mL
5 mL

Used with permission from Pfizer, Inc.

17. medroxyprogesterone 0.9 g

_____

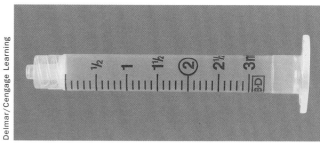

18. gentamicin 70 mg

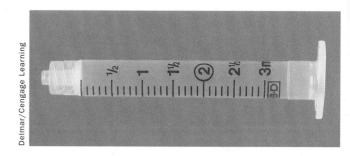

Dosage Ordered   **mL Needed**

19. Vistaril® 120 mg   _____

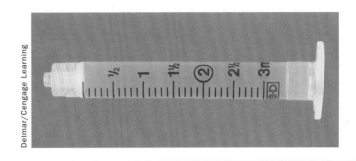

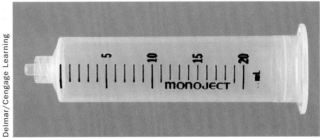

20. sodium chloride 60 mEq for an IV additive   _____

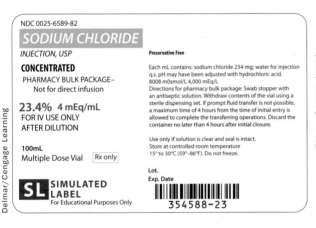

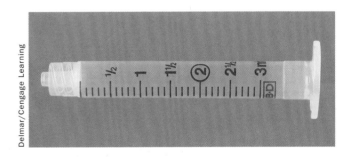

21. atropine sulfate 150 mcg   _____

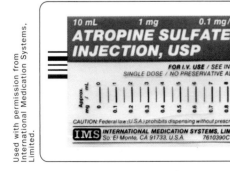

Dosage Ordered

mL Needed

22. meperidine 75 mg

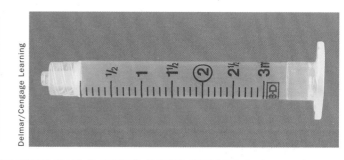

23. fentanyl citrate 80 mcg

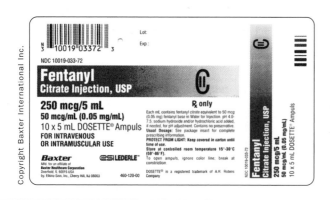

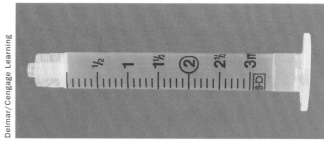

24. celestone 10 mg

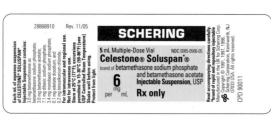

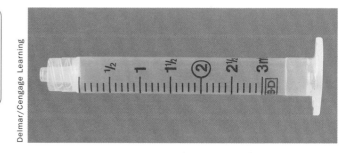

Dosage Ordered   **mL Needed**

25. morphine sulfate 20 mg   _____

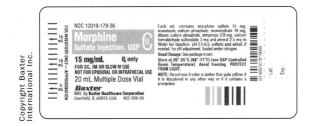
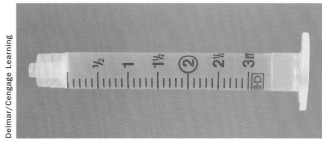

26. gentamicin 0.1 g   _____

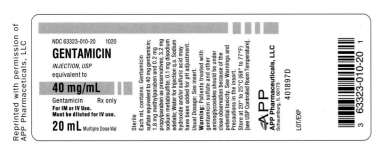
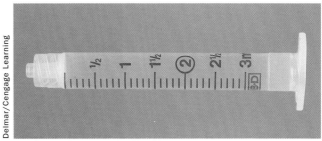

27. Dilantin® 0.15 g   _____

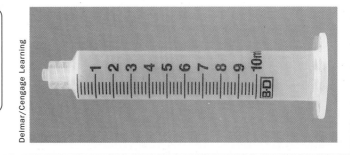

28. doxorubicin HCl 16 mg for an IV additive   _____

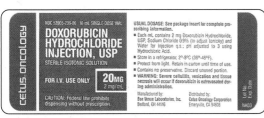

Dosage Ordered   **mL Needed**

29. meperidine HCl 30 mg   _____

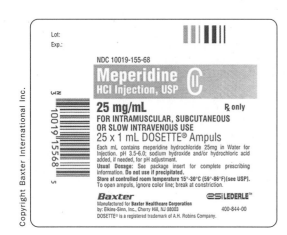

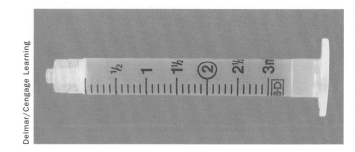

30. methotrexate 40 mg   _____

31. midazolam HCl 3 mg   _____

Dosage Ordered

mL Needed

32. ondansetron 3 mg

_____

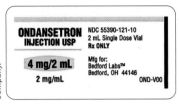

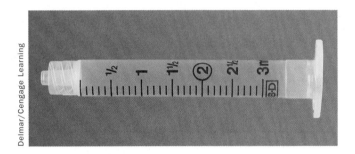

33. dexamethasone 5 mg

_____

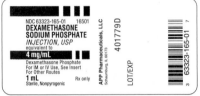

34. hydroxyzine HCl 40 mg

_____

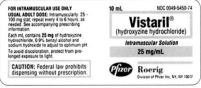

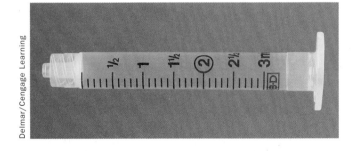

Dosage Ordered

mL Needed

35. Ketorolac tromethamine 20mg

_____

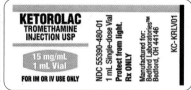

KETOROLAC
TROMETHAMINE
INJECTION USP

15 mg/mL
1 mL Vial

FOR IM OR IV USE ONLY

NDC 55390-480-01
1 mL Single-dose Vial
Protect from light.
Rx ONLY

Manufactured for:
Bedford Laboratories™
Bedford, OH 44146

KC-KRLV01

Delmar/Cengage Learning

36. nalbuphine HCl 30 mg

_____

NDC 63481-509-05

NUBAIN®
(Nalbuphine HCl) Rx only

20 mg/mL injection

10 mL Multiple Dose Vial

Each mL contains: 20 mg nalbuphine HCl, 0.94% sodium citrate hydrous, 1.26% citric acid anhydrous, and 0.2% of a 9:1 mixture of methyl and propylparaben, as preservatives. pH is adjusted, if necessary, to 3.5 to 3.7 with hydrochloric acid.

FOR IM, SC OR IV USE

Usual Dosage: See package insert for complete prescribing information.
Store at 25°C (77°F); excursions permitted to 15°-30°C (59°-86°F).
PROTECT FROM EXCESSIVE LIGHT.

Manufactured for:
Endo Pharmaceuticals Inc.
Chadds Ford, PA 19317

Delmar/Cengage Learning

37. morphine 15 mg

_____

NDC 10019-178-36
Morphine
Sulfate Inj., USP C
10 mg/mL ℞ only
FOR SC, IM OR SLOW IV USE
NOT FOR EPIDURAL OR
INTRATHECAL USE
10 mL Multiple Dose Vial

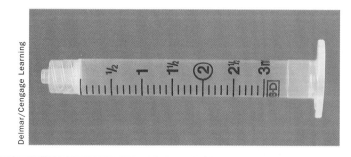

Delmar/Cengage Learning

Dosage Ordered

mL Needed

38. cyanocobalamin 750 mcg

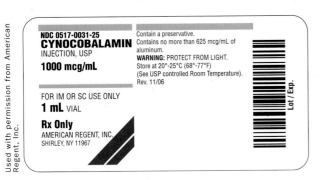

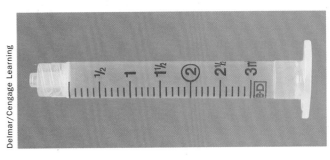

_____

39. aminophylline 0.4 g for an IV additive

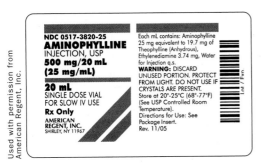

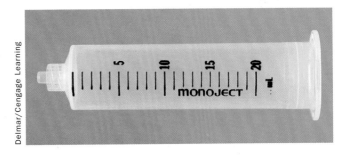

_____

40. Dilantin® 125 mg

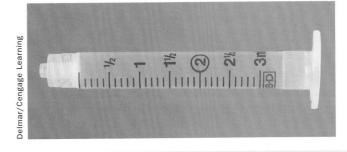

_____

Dosage Ordered   mL Needed

41. Ketorolac 25 mg
_____

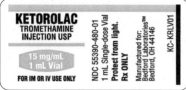

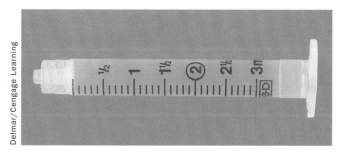

42. Vistaril 50 mg
_____

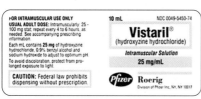

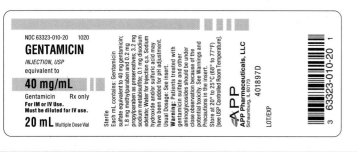

43. gentamicin 0.1 g
_____

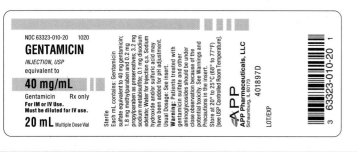

44. Robinul® 180 mcg
_____

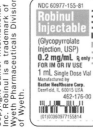

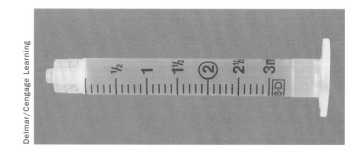

Dosage Ordered   **mL Needed**

45. hydroxyzine HCl 70 mg   _____

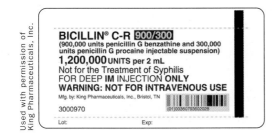 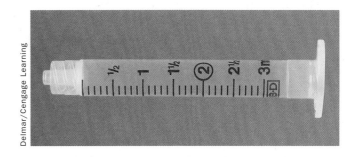

46. Bicillin® C-R 400,000 units   _____

 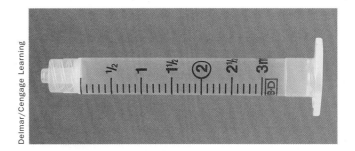

47. heparin sodium 1500 units (calculate to the nearest hundredth)   _____

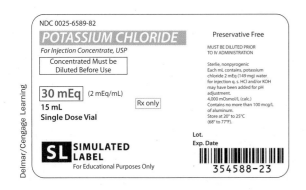 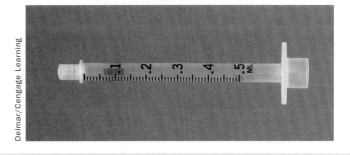

48. potassium chloride 20 mEq for an IV additive   _____

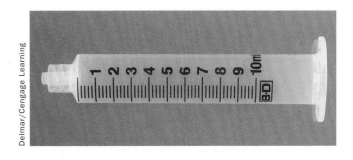

Dosage Ordered

mL Needed

49. Inapsine® 4.5 mg _____

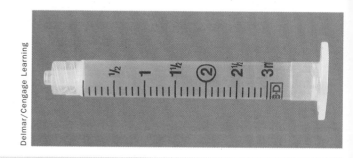

50. epinephrine 1.4 mg _____

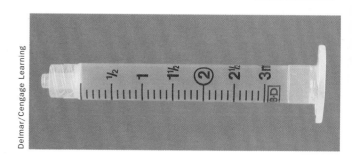

51. Nubain 15 mg _____

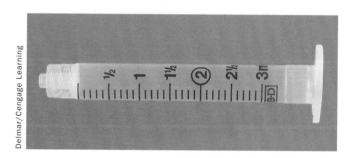

52. furosemide 15 mg _____

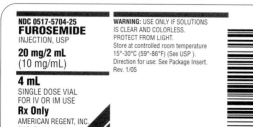

Dosage Ordered   **mL Needed**

53. dexamethasone 6000 mcg   _____

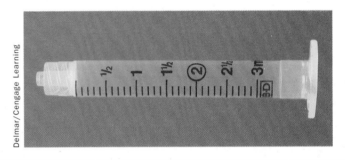

54. phenytoin Na 0.1 g   _____

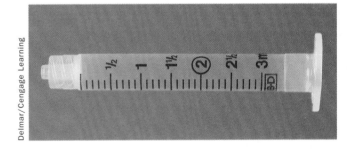

55. lidocaine HCl 15 mg   _____

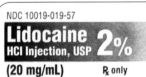

Answers

1. 0.8 mL	**14.** 0.45 mL	**28.** 8 mL	**42.** 2 mL
2. 1.5 mL	**15.** 1.6 mL	**29.** 1.2 mL	**43.** 2 mL
3. 1.4 mL	**16.** 2 mL	**30.** 1.6 mL	**44.** 0.9 mL
4. 3 mL	**17.** 2.3 mL	**31.** 0.6 mL	**45.** 1.4 mL
5. 0.9 mL	**18.** 1.8 mL	**32.** 1.5 mL	**46.** 0.7 mL
6. 1.5 mL	**19.** 2.4 mL	**33.** 1.3 mL	**47.** 0.3 mL
7. 0.38 mL	**20.** 15 mL	**34.** 1.6 mL	**48.** 10 mL
8. 0.8 mL	**21.** 1.5 mL	**35.** 1.3 mL	**49.** 1.8 mL
9. 1.2 mL	**22.** 0.8 mL	**36.** 1.5 mL	**50.** 1.4 mL
10. 0.8 mL	**23.** 1.6 mL	**37.** 1.5 mL	**51.** 0.8 mL
11. 8 mL	**24.** 1.7 mL	**38.** 0.8 mL	**52.** 1.5 mL
12. 2 mL	**25.** 1.3 mL	**39.** 16 mL	**53.** 1.5 mL
13. 1.5 mL	**26.** 2.5 mL	**40.** 2.5 mL	**54.** 2 mL
	27. 3 mL	**41.** 1.7 mL	**55.** 0.8 mL

SECTION 5

Dosage Calculation from Body Weight and Body Surface Area

ADULT AND PEDIATRIC DOSAGES BASED ON BODY WEIGHT

Objectives

The learner will:

1. convert body weight from lb to kg.

2. convert body weight from kg to lb.

3. calculate dosages using mcg/mg per kg, or per lb.

4. determine if dosages ordered are within the normal range.

Body weight is a major factor in calculating drug dosages for both adults and children. It is the **most** important determiner of dosages for infants and neonates, whose ability to metabolize drugs is not fully developed. The dosage that will produce optimum therapeutic results for any particular individual, either child or adult, depends not only on dosage but on individual variables, including drug sensitivities and tolerance, age, weight, sex, and metabolic, pathologic, or psychologic conditions.

The prescriber will order the drug and dosage. However, it is a nursing responsibility to check each dosage to be sure the order is correct. Each drug label or drug package insert provides specific dosage details, but more complete information is readily available in drug formularies, the *PDR*, and other medical references. The hospital pharmacist is the ultimate resource for information.

Individualized dosages may be calculated in terms of mcg or mg per kg or lb per day. The total daily dosage may be administered in divided (more than one) dosages; for example, every 6 hours or every 8 hours.

Because body weight is critical in calculating infant and neonatal dosages, measurement is usually done using a weight scale calibrated in kg. Adult weights may be recorded in either kg or lb, and occasionally, conversions between these two measures are necessary.

CONVERTING LB TO KG

If body weight is recorded in lb, but the drug literature lists dosage per kg, a conversion from lb to kg will be necessary. There are 2.2 lb in 1 kg. This means that **kg body weights are smaller than lb weights**, so **the conversion from lb to kg is made by dividing body weight by 2.2**. For ease of calculation, fractional lb may be converted to the nearest quarter and written as decimal fractions instead of oz: ¼ lb (4 oz) as 0.25, ½ lb (8 oz) as 0.5, and ¾ lb (12 oz) as 0.75. If this kind of accuracy is critical, the prescribing orders should so indicate.

EXAMPLE 1   A child weighs 41 lb 12 oz. Convert to kg.

$$41 \text{ lb } 12 \text{ oz} = 41.75 \div 2.2 = 18.97 = \textbf{19 kg}$$

The kg weight should be a smaller number than 41.75 because you are dividing, and 19 kg is.

EXAMPLE 2   Convert the weight of a 144½ lb adult to kg.

$$144\tfrac{1}{2} \text{ lb} = 144.5 \div 2.2 = 65.68 = \textbf{65.7 kg}$$

EXAMPLE 3   Convert the weight of a 27¼ lb child to kg.

$$27\tfrac{1}{4} \text{ lb} = 27.25 \div 2.2 = 12.38 = \textbf{12.4 kg}$$

Problems 13.1

Convert these body weights. Round to the nearest tenth kg.

1. 58¾ lb = _____ kg
2. 63½ lb = _____ kg
3. 163¼ lb = _____ kg
4. 39¾ lb = _____ kg
5. 100¼ lb = _____ kg

6. 134½ lb = _____ kg
7. 112¾ lb = _____ kg
8. 73¼ lb = _____ kg
9. 121½ lb = _____ kg
10. 92¾ lb = _____ kg

Answers   **1.** 26.7 kg   **2.** 28.9 kg   **3.** 74.2 kg   **4.** 18.1 kg   **5.** 45.6 kg   **6.** 61.1 kg   **7.** 51.3 kg   **8.** 33.3 kg   **9.** 55.2 kg   **10.** 42.2 kg

CONVERTING KG TO LB

There are 2.2 lb in 1 kg. To convert from kg to lb, **multiply by 2.2**. Because you are multiplying, **the answer in lb will be larger than the kg** being converted. Express weight to the nearest tenth lb.

EXAMPLE 1   A child weighs 23.3 kg. Convert to lb.

$$23.3 \text{ kg} = 23.3 \times 2.2 = 51.26 = \textbf{51.3 lb}$$

The answer must be larger because you are multiplying, and it is.

EXAMPLE 2   Convert an adult weight of 73.4 kg to lb.

$$73.4 \text{ kg} = 73.4 \times 2.2 = 161.48 = \textbf{161.5 lb}$$

EXAMPLE 3   Convert the weight of a 14.2 kg child to lb.

$$14.2 \text{ kg} = 14.2 \times 2.2 = 31.24 = \textbf{31.2 lb}$$

Problems 13.2

Convert kg to lb. Round to the nearest tenth lb.

1. 21.3 kg = _____ lb
2. 99.2 kg = _____ lb
3. 28.7 kg = _____ lb
4. 71.4 kg = _____ lb
5. 30.8 kg = _____ lb

6. 43.7 kg = _____ lb
7. 63.8 kg = _____ lb
8. 57.1 kg = _____ lb
9. 84.2 kg = _____ lb
10. 34.9 kg = _____ lb

Answers **1.** 46.9 lb **2.** 218.2 lb **3.** 63.1 lb **4.** 157.1 lb **5.** 67.8 lb **6.** 96.1 lb **7.** 140.4 lb
8. 125.6 lb **9.** 185.2 lb **10.** 76.8 lb

CALCULATING DOSAGES FROM DRUG LABEL INFORMATION

Information you will need to calculate dosages from body weight will be on the actual drug label or on the drug package insert.

Calculating the dosage is a two-step procedure. First, the **total daily dosage** is calculated. Then it is **divided by the number of doses per day** to obtain the actual dose administered at one time.

Let's start by looking at some oral antibiotic labels that contain the mg/kg/day dosage guidelines.

EXAMPLE 1 Refer to the information written sideways on the right of the sample antibiotic label in Figure 13-1 for children's dosages. Notice that the dosage is **20 mg/kg/day (or 40 mg/kg/day in otitis media)**. This dosage is to be given in **divided doses every 8 hours**—or a total of 3 doses (24 hr ÷ 8 hr = 3 doses).

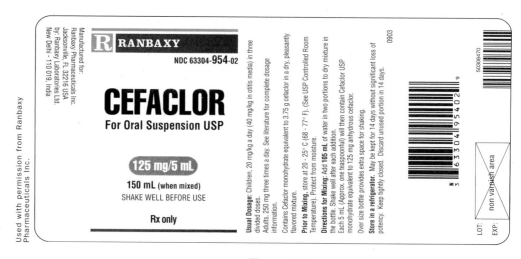

Figure 13-1

Once you have located the dosage information, you can move ahead and calculate the dosage. Let's assume you are checking the dosage ordered for an **18.2 kg** child. Start by calculating the **recommended daily dosage range**.

$$\text{Lower daily dosage} \ = \ \textbf{20 mg/kg}$$

$$20 \text{ mg} \times 18.2 \text{ kg (weight of child)} \ = \ \textbf{364 mg/day}$$

$$\text{Upper daily dosage} \ = \ \textbf{40 mg/kg}$$

$$40 \text{ mg} \times 18.2 \text{ kg} \ = \ \textbf{728 mg/day}$$

The recommended range for this 18.2 kg child is 364–728 mg/day.
The drug is to be given in three divided doses.

$$\textbf{Lower dosage} \quad 364 \text{ mg} \ \div \ 3 \ = \ \textbf{121 mg per dose}$$

$$\textbf{Upper dosage} \quad 728 \text{ mg} \ \div \ 3 \ = \ \textbf{243 mg per dose}$$

The per dose dosage range is 121 mg to 243 mg per dose every 8 hours.

Now that you have the dosage range for this child, you are able to assess the accuracy of physician orders. Let's look at some orders and see how you can use the dosage range you just calculated.

1. **If the order is to give 125 mg every 8 hours, is this within the recommended dosage range?**
   Yes, 125 mg is within the average range of 121–243 mg per dose.

2. **If the order is to give 375 mg every 8 hours, is this within the recommended dosage range?**
   No, this is an overdosage. The maximum recommended dosage is 243 mg per dose. The 375 mg dose should not be given; the prescriber must be called and the order questioned.

3. **If the order is for 75 mg every 8 hours, is this an accurate dosage?**
   The recommended lower limit for an 18.2 kg child is 121 mg. Although 75 mg might be **safe**, it will probably be **ineffective**. Notify the prescriber that the dosage appears to be too low.

4. **If the order is for 250 mg every 8 hours, is this accurate?**
   Because 243 mg per dose is the recommended upper limit, 250 mg is essentially within normal range. The drug strength is 125 mg per 5 mL, and a 250 mg dosage is 10 mL. The prescriber has probably ordered this dosage based on the available dosage strength and for ease of preparation.

5. **If the dosage ordered is 125 mg every 4 hours, is this an accurate dosage?**
   In this order, the **frequency of administration** does not match the recommended dosage of every 8 hours The total daily dosage of 750 mg (125 mg × 6 doses = 750 mg) is slightly, but not significantly, higher than the 728 mg maximum. There may be a reason the prescriber ordered the dosage every 4 hours, but call to verify it.

To determine the safety of an ordered dosage, use body weight to calculate the dosage range ordered, and compare this with the recommended dosage range in mg/kg/day (or mg/lb/day). Assessment must also include the frequency of dosage ordered.

The difference between 4 mg and 6 mg is much more critical than the difference between 243 mg and 250 mg because the drug potency is obviously greater.

Additional factors that must be considered are age, weight, and medical condition. Although these factors cannot be dealt with at length, keep in mind that **the younger, the older, or more compromised by illness an individual is, the more critical a discrepancy is likely to be.**

> Discrepancies in dosages are much more significant if the number of mg or mcg ordered is small.

Problems 13.3

Refer to the Biaxin® Granules label in Figure 13-2 to answer the questions for a 20 lb child.

1. What is the child's body weight in kg to the nearest tenth? _____
2. What is the recommended dosage in mg per day for this child? _____
3. How many mg will this be per dose? _____
4. The order is to give 62.5 mg twice a day. Is this dosage reasonable? _____
5. How many mL would you need to administer this dosage? _____
6. How much water must you add as diluent to prepare this oral suspension? _____

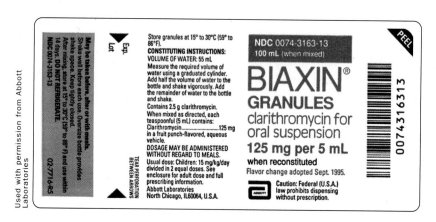

Figure 13-2

Answers   1. 9.1 kg   **2.** 136.5 mg/day   **3.** 68.3 mg/dose   **4.** Yes   **5.** 2.5 mL   **6.** 55 mL

CALCULATING DOSAGES FROM DRUG LITERATURE

The labels you have just been reading were from oral syrups and suspensions, but the same calculation steps are necessary for dosages to be administered by the IV or IM route. Parenteral labels are much smaller in size and usually do not include dosage recommendations. To obtain these, you will have to refer to the **drug package inserts,** the *PDR,* or **similar references**. These references will contain extensive details about each drug's chemistry, actions, adverse reactions, recommended administration, and so on, so it will be necessary for you to search for and select the information you need under the heading **Dosage and Administration.** In the following exercises, the searching has been done for you, and only those excerpts necessary for your calculations are shown.

Problems 13.4

Refer to the cefazolin package insert in Figure 13-3 to locate the information for pediatric dosages.

1. What is the dosage range in mg/kg/day for mild-to-moderate infections? _____

2. What is the dosage range for mild-to-moderate infections in mg/lb/day? _____

3. The total dosage will be divided into how many doses per day? _____

4. In severe infections, what is the maximum daily dosage recommended in mg/kg? _____

   In mg/lb? _____

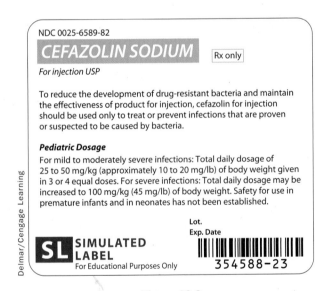

Figure 13-3

Answers   **1.** 25 mg–50 mg   **2.** 10 mg–20 mg   **3.** 3–4 doses per day   **4.** 100 mg/kg; 45 mg/lb

Problems 13.5

Use the information you just obtained from Figure 13-3 to do the calculations for a child who weighs 35 lb and has a moderately severe infection.

1. What is the lower daily dosage range? _____

2. What is the upper daily dosage range? _____

3. If the medication is given in 4 divided dosages, what will the per dosage range be?

_____

4. If a dosage of 125 mg is ordered every 6 hours, will you need to question it?

_____

Answers **1.** 350 mg/day **2.** 700 mg/day **3.** 87.5 mg to 175 mg per dose **4.** No; within normal range

Problems 13.6

Refer to the dosage information in Figure 13-4 to answer the following questions about adult IV dosages.

1. What is the recommended daily dosage range for serious infections?

_____

2. In how many divided doses should this daily dosage be given?

_____

3. What is the maximum daily dosage?

_____

4. Calculate the daily dosage range in g for a 176 lb adult.

_____

5. If this dosage is to be given every 6 hours, what will this individual's dosage range be?

_____

6. If a dosage of 2 g is ordered, what initial assessment would you make about it?

_____

7. If a dosage of 10 g is ordered every 6 hours, what assessment would you make?

_____

DOSAGE AND ADMINISTRATION

MEZLIN® (sterile mezlocillin sodium) may be administered intravenously or intramuscularly. For serious infections, the intravenous route of administration should be used. Intramuscular doses should not exceed 2g per injection.

The recommended adult dosage for serious infections is 200-300 mg/kg per day given in 4 to 6 divided doses. The usual dose is 3g given every 4 hours (18g/day) or 4g given every 6 hours (16g/day). For life-threatening infections, up to 350 mg/kg per day may be administered, but the total daily dosage should ordinarily not exceed 24g.
[See table below.]
For patients with life-threatening infections, 4g may be administered every 4 hours (24g/day).

Used with permission from Novartis AG

Figure 13-4

Answers **1.** 200–300 mg/kg **2.** 4 to 6 doses; every 6 or 4 hours **3.** 24 g **4.** 16–24 g **5.** 4–6 g
6. The dosage is too low **7.** The dosage is too high

Problems 13.7

Refer to the dosage recommendations for the antineoplastic agent in Figure 13-5 to answer the following questions for treatment of testicular tumors in a patient weighing 240 lb.

1. What is the recommended daily dosage range in mcg/kg?   _____

2. How often is this dosage to be given and for how long?   _____   _____

3. What is the daily dosage range in mcg for this patient? In mg? (Calculate kg weight to the nearest tenth.)   _____   _____

4. If a dosage of 3 mg IV is ordered every morning, does this need to be questioned?   _____

MITHRACIN®
(plicamycin)
FOR INTRAVENOUS USE

℞

DOSAGE
The daily dose of Mithracin is based on the patient's body weight. If a patient has abnormal fluid retention such as edema, hydrothorax or ascites, the patient's ideal weight rather than actual body weight should be used to calculate the dose.
Treatment of Testicular Tumors: In the treatment of patients with testicular tumors the recommended daily dose of Mithracin (plicamycin) is 25 to 30 mcg (0.025–0.030 mg) per kilogram of body weight. Therapy should be continued for a period of 8 to 10 days unless significant side effects or toxicity occur during therapy. A course of therapy consisting of more than 10 daily doses is not recommended. Individual daily doses should not exceed 30 mcg (0.030 mg) per kilogram of body weight.

Used with permission of Bayer Corporation

Figure 13-5

Answers   1. 25–30 mcg/kg   **2.** Once a day; 8–10 days   **3.** 2728–3273 mcg/day; 2.7–3.3 mg/day
4. No; within normal range

Problems 13.8

Refer to the Rocephin™ literature in Figure 13-6 to answer the following questions on pediatric dosages.

1. What is the dosage in mg/kg/day for acute bacterial otitis media?   _____

2. What is the dosage range for skin structure infections?   _____

3. What is the initial dosage for meningitis?   _____

4. What will the initial dosage be for a child with meningitis weighing 12.6 kg? In mg? In g?   _____

5. What is the twice-daily dosage in mg for this child to follow the initial dose?   _____

6. What will the initial meningitis dosage be for a child weighting 19½ lb?   _____

7. How many days must rocephin therapy be continued for meningitis after the initial dose?   _____

ROCEPHIN DOSAGE FOR CHILDREN

PEDIATRIC PATIENTS: For the treatment of skin and skin structure infections, the recommended total daily dose is 50 to 75 mg/kg given once a day (or in equally divided doses twice a day). The total daily dose should not exceed 2 grams.

For the treatment of acute bacterial otitis media, a single intramuscular dose of 50 mg/kg (not to exceed 1 gram) is recommended (see **INDICATIONS AND USAGE**).

For the treatment of serious miscellaneous infections other than meningitis, the recommended total daily dose is 50 to 75 mg/kg, given in divided doses every 12 hours. The total daily dose should not exceed 2 grams.

In the treatment of meningitis, it is recommended that the initial therapeutic dose be 100 mg/kg (not to exceed 4 grams). Thereafter, a total daily dose of 100 mg/kg/day (not to exceed 4 grams daily) is recommended. The daily dose may be administered once a day (or in equally divided doses every 12 hours). The usual duration of therapy is 7 to 14 days.

Figure 13-6

Rocephin information is available online at **http://www.rxlist.com/rocephin-drug.htm**.

Answers   **1.** 50 mg/kg   **2.** 50–75 mg/kg once a day or equally divided dosages twice a day   **3.** 100 mg/kg not to exceed 4 g   **4.** 1260 mg; 1.26 g   **5.** 630 mg   **6.** 887 mg   **7.** 7–14 days

Summary

This concludes the chapter on calculation and assessment of dosages based on body weight. The important points to remember from this chapter are:

- Dosages are frequently ordered on the basis of weight, especially for children.

- Dosages may be recommended based on mcg or mg per kg or lb per day, usually administered in divided doses.

- Body weight may need to be converted from kg to lb or lb to kg to correlate with dosage recommendations.

- To convert lb to kg, divide by 2.2; to convert kg to lb, multiply by 2.2.

- Calculating dosage is a two-step procedure: first, calculate the total daily dosage for the weight; then, divide this by the number of doses to be administered.

- To check the accuracy of a prescriber's order, calculate the correct dosage and compare it with the dosage ordered.

- Dosage discrepancies are much more critical if the dosage range is low—for example, 2–5 mg—as opposed to high—for example, 250–500 mg.

- Factors that make discrepancies particularly serious are age, low body weight, and severity of medical condition.

- If the drug label does not contain all the necessary information for safe administration, additional information should be obtained from drug package inserts, the PDR, drug formularies, or the hospital pharmacist.

Summary Self-Test

Read the dosage labels and literature provided to answer the questions.

1. A 43 lb child has an order for oral cefaclor. What is the daily dosage for this child?   _____

2. What is the per dose dosage?   _____

3. Is an order for 250 mg of cefaclor every 8 hours correct for this child?   _____

Used with permission of Ranbaxy Pharmaceuticals Inc.

Manufactured for:
Ranbaxy Pharmaceuticals Inc.
Jacksonville, FL 32216 USA
by: Ranbaxy Laboratories Ltd
New Delhi - 110 019, India

R RANBAXY

NDC 63304-**956**-01

CEFACLOR
For Oral Suspension USP

250 mg/5 mL

75 mL (when mixed)
SHAKE WELL BEFORE USE

Rx only

Usual Dosage: Children, 20 mg/kg a day (40 mg/kg in otitis media) in three divided doses.
Adults, 250 mg three times a day. See literature for complete dosage information.
Contains Cefaclor monohydrate equivalent to 3.75 g cefaclor in a dry, pleasantly flavored mixture.
Prior to Mixing, store at 20 - 25 C (68 - 77 F). (See USP Controlled Room Temperature). Protect from moisture.
Directions for Mixing: Add **53 mL** of water in two portions to dry mixture in the bottle. Shake well after each addition.
Each 5 mL (Approx. one teaspoonful) will then contain Cefaclor USP monohydrate equivalent to 250 mg anhydrous cefaclor.
Over size bottle provides extra space for shaking.
Store in a refrigerator. May be kept for 14 days without significant loss of potency. Keep tightly closed. Discard unused portion in 14 days.

0903

LOT:
EXP:

non varnish area

4. A 140 lb adult has an order for IV methylprednisolone. Calculate this patient's per dose dosage.   _____

5. How often is this dosage to be given?   _____

6. Children's dosages are smaller. What is the lowest mg/kg dosage recommended?   _____

7. Calculate the lowest daily dosage for a child weighing 43 lb.   _____

8. When given intravenously what period of time is specified for the Solu-Medrol administration?   _____

Used with permission of Pfizer Inc.

SOLU–MEDROL®
brand of methylprednisolone sodium succinate sterile powder
(methylprednisolone sodium succinate for injection, USP)
For Intravenous or Intramuscular Administration

DOSAGE AND ADMINISTRATION
When high dose therapy is desired, the recommended dose of SOLU-MEDROL Sterile Powder (methylprednisolone sodium succinate) is 30 mg/kg administered intravenously over at least 30 minutes. This dose may be repeated every 4 to 6 hours for 48 hours.

Dosage may be reduced for infants and children but should be governed more by the severity of the condition and response of the patient than by age or size. It should not be less than 0.5 mg per kg every 24 hours.

9. Refer to the penicillin V potassium oral solution label and identify the dosage strength in mg.   _____

10. What is the dosage strength in units?   _____

11. This medication is shipped in powdered form. How much diluent is needed for reconstitution?   _____

12. What kind of diluent?   _____

13. What dosage in mg/kg is specified for infants?   _____

14. If an infant weighs 6.2 kg, what will the dosage range be?   _____

15. What will the dosage range be for a 16 lb infant?   _____

16. A 7.9 kg infant has an order for 125 mg every 8 hours. Calculate the per dose dosage based on this infant's body weight. Is the penicillin dosage ordered correct?   _____   _____

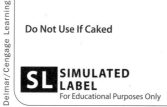

NDC 0025-6589-82

PENICILLIN V POTASSIUM

125 mg (200,000 units)   Rx only
For Oral Solution U.S.P.

**per 5 mL when mixed as directed;
200 mL after mixing**

Contains penicillin V potassium equivalent to 5 grams penicillin V in a dry mixture.

Each 5 mL teaspoon of prepared solution yields penicillin V potassium equivalent to 125 mg (200,000 units) penicillin V.

DIRECTIONS FOR PREPARATION

Use 117 mL of water to prepare 200 mL oral solution. Loosen powder then add water and shake vigorously.
Usual dosage: Adults and children — 1 to 2 teaspoons, given three or four times per day. Infants — 15 to 56 mg/kg body weight daily, given in three to six divided doses. See insert for detailed information.
Store at room temperature in dry form.

Lot.
Exp. Date

Do Not Use If Caked

Delmar/Cengage Learning

SL SIMULATED LABEL
For Educational Purposes Only

354588-23

17. Cefaclor oral suspension has been ordered for a child weighing 100 lb. Calculate the daily dose.   _____

18. What will the per dose dosage be?   _____

19. Would a 5 mL dosage every 8 hours be reasonable for this child?   _____

20. How is this oral cefaclor suspension to be reconstituted?   _____

21. What precautions did you learn about pouring and administering suspensions such as cefaclor?   _____

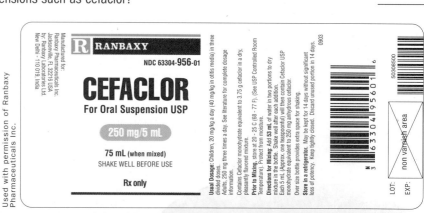

Used with permission of Ranbaxy Pharmaceuticals Inc.

Manufactured for:
Ranbaxy Pharmaceuticals Inc.
Jacksonville, FL 32216 USA
by: Ranbaxy Laboratories Ltd.
New Delhi - 110 019, India

R RANBAXY
NDC 63304-956-01

CEFACLOR
For Oral Suspension USP

250 mg/5 mL

75 mL (when mixed)
SHAKE WELL BEFORE USE

Rx only

Usual Dosage: Children, 20 mg/kg a day (40 mg/kg in otitis media) in three divided doses.
Adults, 250 mg three times a day. See literature for complete dosage information.
Contains Cefaclor monohydrate equivalent to 3.75 g cefaclor in a dry, pleasantly flavored mixture.
Prior to Mixing, store at 20 - 25 C (68 - 77 F). (See USP Controlled Room Temperature). Protect from moisture.
Directions for Mixing: Add 53 mL of water in two portions to dry mixture in the bottle. Shake well after each addition.
Each 5 mL (Approx. one teaspoonful) will then contain Cefaclor USP monohydrate equivalent to 250 mg anhydrous cefaclor.
Over size bottle provides extra space for shaking.
Store in a refrigerator. May be kept for 14 days without significant loss of potency. Keep tightly closed. Discard unused portion in 14 days.

0903

50308500

22. Refer to the acyclovir sodium injection insert to locate the adult and adolescent dosage in mg/kg.

    _____

23. What will the dosage be per dose for an adult with mucosal herpes simplex weighing 61.4 kg?

    _____

24. What would the dosage be for an adolescent with herpes simplex encephalitis weighing 180 lb?

    _____

25. What mg/kg dosage is recommended for an infant with herpes simplex encephalitis?

    _____

26. Read the literature to locate the time period recommended for intravenous infusion.

    _____

27. There are bold print precautions regarding parenteral administration on this insert. What are they?

    _____

ACYCLOVIR SODIUM

INJECTION

DOSAGE AND ADMINISTRATION:
CAUTION - AVOID RAPID OR BOLUS INTRAVENOUS INJECTION. (see WARNINGS and PRECAUTIONS).

AVOID INTRAMUSCULAR OR SUBCUTANEOUS INJECTION (see WARNINGS).
Initiate therapy as early as possible following onset of signs and symptoms of herpes infections.
Do not exceed a dose equivalent to 20 mg/kg every 8 hours for any patient.

DOSAGE IN HERPES SIMPLEX INFECTION:
MUCOSAL AND CUTANEOUS HERPES SIMPLEX (HSV-1 and HSV-2) INFECTIONS IN IMMUNOCOMPROMISED PATIENTS:

Adults and Adolescents 12 years of age and older: 5 mg/kg infused at a constant rate over 1 hour, every 8 hours for 7 days.

Children under 12 years of age: 10 mg/kg infused at a constant rate over 1 hour, every 8 hours for 7 days.

DOSAGE IN SEVERE INITIAL CLINICAL EPISODES OF HERPES GENITALIS:
Adults and Adolescents 12 years of age and older: 5 mg/kg infused at a constant rate over 1 hour, every 8 hours for 5 days.

DOSAGE IN HERPES SIMPLEX ENCEPHALITIS:
Adults and Adolescents 12 years of age and older: 10 mg/kg infused at a constant rate over 1 hour, every 8 hours for 10 days.

Children 3 months to 12 years of age: 20 mg/kg infused at a constant rate over 1 hour, every 8 hours for 10 days.

Administration
Further dilute the calculated dose in an appropriate intravenous solution at a volume selected for administration during each 1 hour infusion. Infusion concentrations of approximately 7 mg/mL or lower are recommended. Clinical studies reveal that the average 70 kg adult received between 60 and 150 mL of fluid per dose. Higher concentrations (e.g.,10 mg/mL) may produce phlebitis or inflammation at the injection site upon inadvertent extravasation. Standard, commercially available electrolyte and glucose solutions are suitable for intravenous administration; biologic or colloidal fluids (e.g., blood products, protein solutions, etc.) are not recommended.
  Once diluted, each dose should be used within 24 hours.
  Visually inspect for particulate matter and discoloration prior to administration, whenever solution and container permit.

354588-23

NDC 0025-6589-82

Delmar/Cengage Learning

SL SIMULATED LABEL
For Educational Purposes Only

Lot.
Exp. Date

---

28. A 198 lb adult is to be treated with IV ticarcillin disodium for bacterial septicemia. What is the daily dosage range in mg for this patient?

    _____

29. If the drug is administered every 4 hours, what will the per dose be in g?

    _____

30. Do you need to question a per dose dosage of 4 g of ticarcillin every 4 hours for this patient?

    _____

TICARCILLIN DISODIUM

FOR INTRAMUSCULAR OR INTRAVENOUS ADMINISTRATION

DOSAGE AND ADMINISTRATION
In serious urinary tract and systemic infections, intravenous therapy in the higher doses should be used. Intramuscular injections should not exceed 2 grams per injection.

Adults:

Bacterial septicemia	200 to 300 mg/kg/day by I.V. infusion in divided doses every four or six hours.
Respiratory tract infection	Usual dose is 3 grams every four hours (18 grams/day) or 4 grams every six hours
Skin and soft-tissue infection	(16 grams/day) depending on weight and the severity of the infection.
Intra-abdominal infection	
Infections of the female pelvis and genital tract	

Urinary tract infections	
Complicated:	Give 150 to 200 mg/kg/day by I.V. infusion every four to six hours in divided doses. Recommended dosage for average (70 kg) adult: 3 grams four times daily.
Uncomplicated:	Give 1 gram I.M. or direct I.V. every six hours.

SL SIMULATED LABEL
For Educational Purposes Only

Delmar/Cengage Learning

354588-23

NDC 0025-6589-82

Lot.
Exp. Date

31. Refer to the VFEND® package insert information to locate the IV maintenance dosage in mg/kg every 12 hours (written with the abbreviation q12h, now slated for deletion) for invasive aspergillosis. _____

32. What would the daily IV dosage be for an individual weighing 92.7 kg? _____

33. What would the daily oral dosage be for this same 92.7 kg individual? _____

34. What will a single IV maintenance dosage be for the same 92.7 kg individual? _____

35. Locate the VFEND information on the maximum rate of administration for intravenous administration. _____

36. There is a bold type and capitalized warning for IV administration of VFEND on this insert. What is it? _____

VFEND® I.V.

(voriconazole) for Injection

VFEND® Tablets

(voriconazole)

VFEND® (voriconazole) for Oral Suspension

DESCRIPTION
VFEND® (voriconazole), a triazole antifungal agent, is available as a lyophilized powder for solution for intravenous infusion, film-coated tablets for oral administration, and as a powder for oral suspension.

DOSAGE AND ADMINISTRATION

Administration
VFEND Tablets or Oral Suspension should be taken at least one hour before, or one hour following, a meal.

VFEND I.V. for Injection requires reconstitution to 10 mg/mL and subsequent dilution to 5 mg/mL or less prior to administration as an infusion, at a maximum rate of 3 mg/kg per hour over 1–2 hours (see Intravenous Administration).
NOT FOR IV BOLUS INJECTION

Recommended Dosing Regimen

| Infection | Loading dose | Maintenance Dose | |
	IV	IV	Oral[a]
Invasive Aspergillosis	6 mg/kg q12h for the first 24 hours	4 mg/kg q12h	200 mg q12h
Candidemia in nonneutropenic patients and other deep tissue *Candida* infections	6 mg/kg q12h for the first 24 hours	3–4 mg/kg q12h[b]	200 mg q12h
Esophageal Candidiasis	c	c	200 mg q12h
Scedosporiosis and Fusariosis	6 mg/kg q12h for the first 24 hours	4 mg/kg q12h	200 mg q12h

Used with permission of Pfizer Inc.

FZC-P01

FLUCONAZOLE INJECTION

For Intravenous Infusion Only
Rx ONLY
DESCRIPTION

Fluconazole, the first of a new subclass of synthetic triazole antifungal agents, is available as a sterile solution for intravenous use in glass vials.

Dosage and Administration in Children:

The following dose equivalency scheme should generally provide equivalent exposure in pediatric and adult patients:

Pediatric Patients	Adults
3 mg/kg	100 mg
6 mg/kg	200 mg
12*mg/kg	400 mg

*Some older children may have clearances similar to that of adults. Absolute doses exceeding 600 mg/day are not recommended. Experience with fluconazole in neonates is limited to pharmacokinetic studies in premature newborns. (See **CLINICAL PHARMACOLOGY.**) Based on the prolonged half-life seen in premature newborns (gestational age 26 to 29 weeks), these children, in the first two weeks of life, should receive the same dosage (mg/kg) as in older children, but administered every 72 hours. After the first two weeks, these children should be dosed once daily. No information regarding fluconazole pharmacokinetics in full-term newborns is available.

Oropharyngeal candidiasis: The recommended dosage of fluconazole for oropharyngeal candidiasis in children is 6 mg/kg on the first day, followed by 3 mg/kg once daily. Treatment should be administered for at least 2 weeks to decrease the likelihood of relapse.

Esophageal candidiasis: For the treatment of esophageal candidiasis, the recommended dosage of fluconazole in children is 6 mg/kg on the first day, followed by 3 mg/kg once daily. Doses up to 12 mg/kg/day may be used based on medical judgment of the patient's response to therapy. Patients with esophageal candidiasis should be treated for a minimum of three weeks and for at least 2 weeks following the resolution of symptoms.

Systemic Candida infections: For the treatment of candidemia and disseminated *Candida* infections, daily doses of 6 to 12 mg/kg/day have been used in an open, noncomparative study of a small number of children.

Cryptococcal meningitis: For the treatment of acute cryptococcal meningitis, the recommended dosage is 12 mg/kg on the first day, followed by 6 mg/kg once daily. A dosage of 12 mg/kg once daily may be used, based on medical judgment of the patient's response to therapy. The recommended duration of treatment for initial therapy of cryptococcal meningitis is 10 to 12 weeks after the cerebrospinal fluid becomes culture negative. For suppression of relapse of cryptococcal meningitis in children with AIDS, the recommended dose of fluconazole is 6 mg/kg once daily.

37. Refer to the fluconazole injection insert to locate the first day dosage for a child with esophageal candidiasis.   _____

38. What is the dosage recommendation for subsequent days?   _____

39. How long must treatment for this condition be continued?   _____

40. What will the first dose be for a child weighing 18.2 kg?   _____

41. What will the subsequent dosage be for this same 18.2 kg child?   _____

42. How often will this dosage be administered?   _____

43. What is the maximum mg/kg dosage recommended if the child has a particularly severe infection?   _____

44. What would the first dose of fluconazole be for a child weighing 72 lb?   _____

Answers

1. 390 mg
2. 130 mg/dose
3. No, too high
4. 1908 mg/dose
5. Every 4 to 6 hours for 48 hours
6. 0.5 mg/kg every 24 hours
7. 9.8 mg/day
8. At least 30 minutes
9. 125 mg/5 mL
10. 200,000 units/ 5 mL
11. 117 mL
12. Water
13. 15–56 mg/kg
14. 93–347 mg
15. 110–409 mg/daily
16. 40–147 mg/dose; the 125 ordered is correct
17. 910 mg/day
18. 303 mg/dose
19. Yes
20. Add 53 mL water in 2 portions. Shake well after each addition until mixed.
21. Shake well to mix completely before pouring; administer immediately to prevent settling out.
22. 5 mg/kg
23. 307 mg
24. 818 mg
25. 20 mg/kg
26. 1 hour
27. No rapid or bolus injection; no intramuscular or subcutaneous injection
28. 18,000–27,000 mg daily
29. 3–4.5 g/dose
30. No
31. 4 mg/kg
32. 742 mg daily
33. 400 mg daily
34. 371 mg/dose
35. 3 mg/kg per hour over 1–2 hours
36. Not for IV bolus injection
37. 6 mg/kg
38. 3 mg/kg
39. Minimum of three weeks and at least two weeks following resolution of symptoms
40. 109 mg
41. 55 mg
42. Once daily
43. 12 mg/kg/day
44. 196 mg

ADULT AND PEDIATRIC DOSAGES BASED ON BODY SURFACE AREA

Body surface area (BSA or SA) is a major factor in calculating dosages for a number of drugs, because many of the body's physiologic processes are more closely related to body surface than they are to weight. Body surface is used extensively to calculate dosages of antineoplastic agents for cancer chemotherapy, and for patients with severe burns. However, an increasing number of other drugs is also calculated using BSA. The nursing responsibility for checking dosages based on BSA varies widely in clinical facilities; therefore, this chapter covers all three essentials: calculation of BSA, calculation of dosages based on BSA, and assessment of physician orders based on BSA.

Body surface is calculated in **square meters (m²)** using the patient's **weight and height** and a calculator that has **square root (√)** capabilities. Two formulas are used by physicians and pharmacists: one using kg and cm measurements, and another using lb (pound) and in (inch) measurements. We'll look at these separately.

CALCULATING BSA FROM kg AND cm

The safest way to calculate BSA is by using a time-tested formula with kilogram and centimeter measurements.

$$\text{BSA} = \sqrt{\frac{\text{wt(kg)} \times \text{ht(cm)}}{3600}}$$

Objectives

The learner will:

1. calculate BSA using formulas for weight and height.

2. use BSA to calculate dosages.

3. assess the accuracy of dosages prescribed on the basis of BSA.

EXAMPLE 1   Calculate the BSA of a man who weighs **104 kg** and whose height is **191 cm**. Express BSA to the nearest hundredth.

$$\sqrt{\frac{104(\text{kg}) \times 191(\text{cm})}{3600}}$$

$$= \sqrt{5.517}$$

$$= 2.348 = \textbf{2.35 m}^2$$

Calculators vary in the way a square root must be obtained. Here is how the BSA was calculated in this example and throughout the chapter:

$$104. \times 191. \div 3600. = 5.517, \text{ then immediately enter } \sqrt{}$$

Practice with your own calculator to determine how to calculate a square root. Be careful to **insert periods after all whole numbers** or you may obtain a wrong answer from preset decimal placement.

   The m^2 **BSA is rounded to hundredths**. Answers may vary slightly depending on how your calculator is set. Consider answers within 2–3 hundredths correct. Fractional weights and heights are also used in calculations. Refer to Examples 2 and 3.

EXAMPLE 2   Calculate the BSA of an adolescent who weighs **59.1 kg** and is **157.5 cm** in height. Express BSA to the nearest hundredth.

$$\sqrt{\frac{59.1(\text{kg}) \times 157.5(\text{cm})}{3600}}$$

$$= \sqrt{2.585}$$

$$= 1.607 = \textbf{1.61 m}^2$$

EXAMPLE 3   A child is **96.2 cm** tall and weighs **15.17 kg**. What is his BSA in m^2 to the nearest hundredth?

$$\sqrt{\frac{15.17(\text{kg}) \times 96.2(\text{cm})}{3600}}$$

$$= \sqrt{0.4053}$$

$$= 0.636 = \textbf{0.63 m}^2$$

Problems 14.1

Calculate the BSA in m². Express answers to the nearest hundredth.

1. An adult weighing 59 kg whose height is 160 cm.   _____

2. A child weighing 35.9 kg whose height is 63.5 cm.   _____

3. A child weighing 7.7 kg whose height is 40 cm.   _____

4. An adult weighing 92 kg whose height is 178 cm. _____
5. A child weighing 46 kg whose height is 102 cm. _____

Answers   1. 1.62 m² **2.** 0.8 m² **3.** 0.29 m² **4.** 2.13 m² **5.** 1.14 m²

CALCULATING BSA FROM lb AND in

The formula for calculating BSA from lb and in measurements is equally easy to use. **The only difference is the denominator, which is 3131.**

$$BSA = \sqrt{\frac{wt(lb) \times ht(in)}{3131}}$$

EXAMPLE 1   Calculate BSA to the nearest hundredth for a child who is **24 in** tall and weighs **34 lb**.

$$\sqrt{\frac{34(lb) \times 24(in)}{3131}}$$

$$= \sqrt{0.260}$$

$$= 0.510 = \mathbf{0.51\ m^2}$$

EXAMPLE 2   Calculate BSA to the nearest hundredth for an adult who is **61.3 in** tall and weighs **142.7 lb**.

$$\sqrt{\frac{142.7(lb) \times 61.3(in)}{3131}}$$

$$= \sqrt{2.793}$$

$$= 1.671 = \mathbf{1.67\ m^2}$$

EXAMPLE 3   A child weighs **105 lb** and is **51 in** tall. Calculate BSA to the nearest hundredth.

$$\sqrt{\frac{105(lb) \times 51(in)}{3131}}$$

$$= \sqrt{1.710}$$

$$= 1.307 = \mathbf{1.31\ m^2}$$

Problems 14.2

Determine the BSA. Express answers to the nearest hundredth.

1. A child weighing 92 lb who measures 35 in. _____
2. An adult who weighs 175 lb and who is 67 in tall. _____
3. An adult who is 70 in tall and weighs 194 lb. _____

4. A child who weighs 72.4 lb and is 40.5 in tall. _____

5. A child who measures 26 in and weighs 36 lb. _____

Answers   **1.** 1.01 m²   **2.** 1.94 m²   **3.** 2.08 m²   **4.** 0.97 m²   **5.** 0.55 m²

DOSAGE CALCULATION BASED ON BSA

Once you know the BSA in m², dosage calculation is straight multiplication.

EXAMPLE 1   Dosage recommended is **5 mg per m²**. The child has a BSA of **1.1 m²**.

$1.1(m^2) \times 5\,mg = \textbf{5.5 mg}$

EXAMPLE 2   The recommended child's dosage is 25–50 mg/m². The child has a BSA of **0.76 m²**.

Lower dosage $0.76(m^2) \times 25\,mg = 19\,mg$

Upper dosage $0.76(m^2) \times 50\,mg = 38\,mg$

The dosage range is 19–38 mg.

Problems 14.3

Determine the dosage for the following drugs. Express answers to the nearest whole number.

1. The recommended child's dosage is 5–10 mg/m². The BSA is 0.43 m². _____

2. A child with a BSA of 0.81 m² is to receive a drug with a recommended dosage of 40 mg/m². _____

3. Calculate the recommended dosage of 20 mg/m² for a child with a BSA of 0.51 m². _____

4. An adult is to receive a drug with a recommended dosage of 20–40 units/m². The BSA is 1.93 m². _____

5. The adult recommended dosage is 3–5 mg/m². Calculate dosage for 2.08 m². _____

Answers   **1.** 2–4 mg   **2.** 32 mg   **3.** 10 mg   **4.** 39–77 units   **5.** 6–10 mg

ASSESSING ORDERS BASED ON BSA

In situations where you will have to check a dosage against m² recommendations, you will be referring to drug package inserts, medication protocols, or the *Physicians' Desk Reference* (*PDR*) to determine what the dosage should be.

EXAMPLE 1   Refer to the vinblastine information insert in Figure 14-1 and calculate the **first dose** for an adult whose BSA is **1.66 m²**. Calculations are to the nearest whole number.

Recommended first dose $= 3.7 \text{ mg/m}^2$

$1.66(\text{m}^2) \times 3.7 \text{ mg} = 6.14 = \textbf{6 mg}$

EXAMPLE 2   A child with a BSA of 0.96 m² is to receive her **fourth dose** of vinblastine.

Recommended fourth dose $= 6.25 \text{ mg/m}^2$

$0.96(\text{m}^2) \times 6.25 \text{ mg} = \textbf{6 mg}$

cetus oncology

STERILE VINBLASTINE SULFATE, USP

DOSAGE AND ADMINISTRATION

Caution: It is extremely important that the needle be properly positioned in the vein before this product is injected.

If leakage into surrounding tissue should occur during intravenous administration of vinblastine sulfate, it may cause considerable irritation. The injection should be discontinued immediately, and any remaining portion of the dose should then be introduced into another vein. Local injection of hyaluronidase and the application of moderate heat to the area of leakage help disperse the drug and are thought to minimize discomfort and the possibility of cellulitis.

There are variations in the depth of the leukopenic response which follows therapy with vinblastine sulfate. For this reason, it is recommended that the drug be given no more frequently than *once every 7 days*. It is wise to initiate therapy for adults by administering a single intravenous dose of 3.7 mg/M² of body surface area (bsa); the initial dose for children should be 2.5 mg/M². Thereafter, white-blood-cell counts should be made to determine the patient's sensitivity to vinblastine sulfate. A reduction of 50% in the dose of vinblastine is recommended for patients having a direct serum bilirubin value above 3 mg/100 mL. Since metabolism and excretion are primarily hepatic, no modification is recommended for patients with impaired renal function.

A simplified and conservative incremental approach to dosage *at weekly intervals* may be outlined as follows:

	Adults		Children	
First dose	3.7	mg/M² bsa	2.5	mg/M² bsa
Second dose	5.5	mg/M² bsa	3.75	mg/M² bsa
Third dose	7.4	mg/M² bsa	5	mg/M² bsa
Fourth dose	9.25	mg/M² bsa	6.25	mg/M² bsa
Fifth dose	11.1	mg/M² bsa	7.5	mg/M² bsa

The above-mentioned increases may be used until a maximum dose (not exceeding 18.5 mg/M² bsa for adults and 12.5 mg/M² bsa for children) is reached. The dose should not be increased after that dose which reduces the white-cell count to approximately 3000 cells/mm³. In some adults, 3.7 mg/M² bsa may produce this leukopenia; other adults may require more than 11.1mg/M² bsa; and, very rarely, as much as 18.5 mg/M² bsa may be necessary. For most adult patients, however, the weekly dosage will prove to be 5.5 to 7.4 mg/M² bsa.

Figure 14-1

Problems 14.4

Calculate the following dosages of vinblastine to the nearest whole number from the information available in Figure 14-1.

1. Calculate the dosage for an adult's third dose.
   The patient's BSA is 1.91 m². _____

2. Calculate the child's first dosage for a patient with a
   BSA of 1.2 m². _____

3. Calculate the adult's fifth dosage. The BSA is 1.53 m². _____

4. Calculate the child's second dosage for a BSA of 1.01 m². _____

5. Calculate the adult's second dose for a BSA of 2.12 m². _____

Answers **1.** 14 mg **2.** 3 mg **3.** 17 mg **4.** 4 mg **5.** 12 mg

Problems 14.5

Refer to Figure 14-2 for BiCNU® to locate the following information. Express all dosages to the nearest whole number.

1. What is the dosage per m² if the drug is to be given
   in a single dose? _____

2. If the patient has a BSA of 1.91 m², what will the daily dosage
   range be? _____

3. If the order for this patient is a single dosage of 325 mg,
   is there any need to question it? _____

4. If the dosage ordered is 450 mg, is there any need to
   question it? _____

BiCNU ®
(carmustine for injection)

DOSAGE AND ADMINISTRATION
The recommended dose of BiCNU as a single agent in previously un-treated patients is 150 to 200 mg/m² intravenously every 6 weeks. This may be given as a single dose or divided into daily injections such as 75 to 100 mg/m² on 2 successive days. When BiCNU is used in combination with other myelosuppressive drugs or in patients in whom bone marrow reserve is depleted, the doses should be adjusted accordingly.

Figure 14-2

Answers **1.** 150–200 mg/m² **2.** 287–382 mg **3.** No **4.** Yes, too high

Problems 14.6

Refer to the package insert for the antineoplastic medication bleomycin in Figure 14-3 to answer the following questions.

1. Locate the dosage information on Hodgkin's disease and identify the dosage per m². _____

2. This insert also identifies the dosage per kg. What is this dosage? _____

3. Calculate the unit dosage based on m² for an adult with a BSA of 1.73 m². _____

4. How often is dosage recommended? _____

BLEOMYCIN FOR INJECTION USP
Rx ONLY

BLE-P03

To reduce the development of drug-resistant bacteria and maintain the effectiveness of bleomycin and other antibacterial drugs, bleomycin should be used only to treat or prevent infections that are proven or strongly suspected to be caused by bacteria.

WARNING

It is recommended that bleomycin be administered under the supervision of a qualified physician experienced in the use of cancer chemotherapeutic agents. Appropriate management of therapy and complications is possible only when adequate diagnostic and treatment facilities are readily available.

Pulmonary fibrosis is the most severe toxicity associated with bleomycin. The most frequent presentation is pneumonitis occasionally progressing to pulmonary fibrosis. Its occurrence is higher in elderly patients and in those receiving greater than 400 units total dose, but pulmonary toxicity has been observed in young patients and those treated with low doses.

A severe idiosyncratic reaction consisting of hypotension, mental confusion, fever, chills, and wheezing has been reported in approximately 1% of lymphoma patients treated with bleomycin.

DOSAGE AND ADMINISTRATION

Because of the possibility of an anaphylactoid reaction, lymphoma patients should be treated with 2 units or less for the first two doses. If no acute reaction occurs, then the regular dosage schedule may be followed.

The following dose schedule is recommended:

Squamous cell carcinoma, non-Hodgkin's lymphoma, testicular carcinoma—0.25 to 0.50 units/kg (10 to 20 units/m²) given intravenously, intramuscularly, or subcutaneously weekly or twice weekly.

Hodgkin's Disease—0.25 to 0.50 units/kg (10 to 20 units/m²) given intravenously, intramuscularly, or subcutaneously weekly or twice weekly. After a 50% response, a maintenance dose of 1 unit daily or 5 units weekly intravenously or intramuscularly should be given.

Pulmonary toxicity of bleomycin appears to be dose related with a striking increase when the total dose is over 400 units. Total doses over 400 units should be given with great caution. **Note: When bleomycin for injection is used in combination with other antineoplastic agents, pulmonary toxicities may occur at lower doses.**

Improvement of Hodgkin's Disease and testicular tumors is prompt and noted within 2 weeks. If no improvement is seen by this time, improvement is unlikely Squamous cell cancers respond more slowly, sometimes requiring as long as 3 weeks before any improvement is noted.

Malignant Pleural Effusion—60 units administered as a single dose bolus intrapleural injection (see **Administration: Intrapleural**).

Figure 14-3

Answers 1. 10–20 units/m² **2.** 0.25 to 0.5 units/kg **3.** 17–35 units **4.** Weekly or twice weekly

Problems 14.7

Refer to the mitomycin package insert information in Figure 14-4 to answer the following questions.

1. This preparation is a combination of two different drugs. It is shipped in powdered form. How much diluent must be added to prepare a mitomycin 40 mg and mannitol 80 mg dosage strength? _____

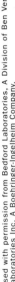

2. What kind of diluent is specified? _____

3. What dosage is required in m²? _____

4. What mitomycin dosage will be required for an individual with a BSA of 1.73? _____

5. How will this be administered? _____

BEDFORD LABORATORIES™

MITOMYCIN FOR INJECTION, USP

Rx ONLY.

DOSAGE AND ADMINISTRATION

Mitomycin should be given intravenously only, using care to avoid extravasation of the compound. If extravasation occurs, cellulitis, ulceration, and slough may result.

Each vial contains either mitomycin 5 mg and mannitol 10 mg, or mitomycin 20 mg and mannitol 40 mg, or mitomycin 40 mg and mannitol 80 mg. To administer, add Sterile Water for Injection, 10 mL 40 mL, or 80 mL, respectively. Shake to dissolve. If product does not dissolve immediately, allow to stand at room temperature until solution is obtained.

After full hematological recovery (see guide to dosage adjustment) from any previous chemotherapy, the following dosage schedule may be used at 6- to 8-week intervals:

20 mg/m² intravenously as a single dose via a functioning intravenous catheter.

Because of cumulative myelosuppression, patients should be fully reevaluated after each course of mitomycin, and the dose reduced if the patient has experienced any toxicities. Doses greater than 20 mg/m² have not been shown to be more effective and are more toxic than lower doses.

Figure 14-4

Answers **1.** 80 mL **2.** Sterile Water for Injection **3.** mitomycin 20 mg/m² **4.** 35 mg
5. Intravenously as a single dose via a functioning intravenous catheter

Summary

This concludes the chapter on dosage calculation based on BSA. The important points to remember from this chapter are:

- The BSA in m² is calculated from a patient's weight and height.

- BSA is more important than weight alone in calculating some drug dosages because many physiologic processes are more closely related to surface area than they are to weight.

- BSA is calculated in square meters (m²) using a formula.

- Two formulas for calculation of BSA are available:

Using kg and cm: $\sqrt{\dfrac{wt(kg) \times ht(cm)}{3600}}$ Using lb and in: $\sqrt{\dfrac{wt(lb) \times ht(in)}{3131}}$

- After the BSA has been obtained, it can be used to calculate specific drug dosages and assess accuracy of physician orders.

Summary Self-Test

Use the formula method to calculate the following BSAs. Express m² to the nearest hundredth.

1. The weight is 58 lb and the height is 36 in.　　　　　_____

2. An adult weighing 74 kg and measuring 160 cm.　　_____

3. A child who is 14.2 kg and measures 64 cm.　　　　_____

4. An adult weighing 69 kg whose height is 170 cm.　　_____

5. An adolescent who is 55 in and 103 lb.　　　　　　_____

6. A child who is 112 cm and weighs 25.3 kg.　　　　_____

7. An adult who weighs 55 kg and measures 157.5 cm.　_____

8. An adult who weighs 65.4 kg and is 132 cm in height.　_____

9. A child whose height is 58 in and whose weight is 26.5 lb.　_____

10. A child whose height is 60 cm and weight is 13.6 kg.　_____

Read the drug insert information provided in Figure 14-5 to answer the following questions. Calculate dosages to the nearest whole number.

11. Read the information on children's dosage to calculate the daily dosage for a 6-year-old child whose BSA is 0.78 m². 　　　　　_____

12. If a dosage of 4 mg is ordered for this 6-year-old child, would you question it? 　　　　_____

13. What would the daily dosage be for a 4-year-old child whose BSA is 0.29 m²? 　　　_____

14. What would the daily dosage be for a 5-year-old child with a BSA of 0.51 m²? 　　　_____

Antibiotic

DOSAGE AND ADMINISTRATION

　DOSAGE SHOULD BE INDIVIDUALIZED ACCORDING TO THE NEEDS AND THE RESPONSE OF THE PATIENT.
　Each tablet contains 4 mg of antibiotic.

Pediatric Patients

Age 2 to 6 years
　The total daily dosage for pediatric patients may be calculated on the basis of body weight or body area using approximately 0.25 mg/kg/day or 8 mg per square meter of body surface (8 mg/m²).
　The usual dose is 2 mg (½ tablet) two or three times a day, adjusted as necessary to the size and response of the patient. The dose is not to exceed 12 mg a day.

Age 7 to 14 years
　The usual dose is 4 mg (1 tablet) two or three times a day, adjusted as necessary to the size and response of the patient. The dose is not to exceed 16 mg a day.

Adults
　The total daily dose for adults should not exceed 0.5 mg/kg/day.
　The therapeutic range is 4 to 20 mg a day, with the majority of patients requiring 12 to 16 mg a day. An occasional patient may require as much as 32 mg a day for adequate relief. It is suggested that dosage be initiated with 4 mg (1 tablet) three times a day and adjusted according to the size and response of the patient.

Delmar/Cengage Learning.

Figure 14-5

Refer to Figure 14-6 to answer the following questions.

15. A patient is to be treated with the drug carboplatin for ovarian carcinoma. Her BSA is 1.61 m². What will her dosage be? _____

16. Another patient with ovarian cancer, who weighs 130 lb and measures 62 in, is to receive carboplatin. What is her BSA? _____

17. What dosage of carboplatin will she require? _____

18. Carboplatin is given in conjunction with cyclophosphamide. What is the recommended m² dosage for this drug? _____

19. Calculate the BSA of a third patient who is receiving therapy for ovarian cancer. She weighs 53.2 kg and measures 150.3 cm. _____

20. What will the companion dosage of cyclophosphamide be for this patient? _____

Manufactured by:
Ben Venue Laboratories, Inc.
Bedford, OH 44146

Manufactured for:
Bedford Laboratories™
Bedford, OH 44146

Patient Information
CARBOplatin for Injection

Read this entire leaflet carefully.
Keep it for future reference.

This information will help you learn more about CARBOplatin for Injection. It cannot, however, cover all the possible warnings or side effects relating to CARBOplatin, and it does not list all of the benefits and risks of CARBOplatin. Your doctor should always be your first choice for detailed information about your medical condition and your treatment. Be sure to ask your doctor about any questions you may have.

DOSAGE AND ADMINISTRATION

NOTE: Aluminum reacts with carboplatin causing precipitate formation and loss of potency, therefore, needles or intravenous sets containing aluminum parts that may come in contact with the drug must not be used for the preparation or administration of carboplatin.

Single Agent Therapy

Carboplatin for injection, as a single agent, has been shown to be effective in patients with recurrent ovarian carcinoma at a dosage of 360 mg/m² IV on day 1 every 4 weeks (alternatively see **Formula Dosing**). In general, however, single intermittent courses of carboplatin should not be repeated until the neutrophil count is at least 2000 and the platelet count is at least 100,000.

Combination Therapy with Cyclophosphamide

In the chemotherapy of advanced ovarian cancer, an effective combination for previously untreated patients consists of:
Carboplatin injection—300 mg/m² IV on day 1 every four weeks for six cycles (alternatively see **Formula Dosing**).
Cyclophosphamide—600 mg/m² IV on day 1 every four weeks for six cycles. For directions regarding the use and administration of cyclophosphamide please refer to its package insert. (See **CLINICAL STUDIES**.)

Figure 14-6

Answers

1. 0.82 m²	**6.** 0.89 m²	**12.** Yes; too low	**18.** 600 mg
2. 1.81 m²	**7.** 1.55 m²	**13.** 2 mg per day	**19.** 1.49 m²
3. 0.50 m²	**8.** 1.55 m²	**14.** 4 mg	**20.** 894 mg
4. 1.81 m²	**9.** 0.70 m²	**15.** 580 mg	
5. 1.35 m²	**10.** 0.48 m²	**16.** 1.6 m²	
	11. 6 mg per day	**17.** 576 mg	

15

INTRODUCTION TO IV THERAPY

Objectives

The learner will:

1. differentiate between primary, secondary, peripheral, and central IV lines.

2. explain the function of IV drip chambers, roller and slide clamps, and on-line and indwelling injection ports.

3. differentiate between heparin flush and heparin admixture dosage strengths.

4. differentiate between volumetric pumps, syringe pumps, and PCAs.

5. identify the abbreviations used for IV fluid orders.

The calculations associated with IV therapy will be easier to understand if you have some general understanding of IV therapy. Intravenous fluid and medication administration is one of the most challenging of all nursing responsibilities. There are currently estimated to be over 200 different manufactured IV fluids, and at least as many additives are used with IV fluids, including medications, electrolytes, and nutrients. In addition, there are hundreds of different types of IV administration sets and components, and dozens of different models of electronic infusion devices (EIDs) to infuse and monitor IV fluids. This would appear to make the entire subject of IV therapy overwhelming, but it is not. This chapter presents the essentials in understandable segments and will provide you with an excellent base of instruction upon which to build. Let's begin by looking at a basic sterile IV setup, which is referred to as a primary line.

PRIMARY LINE

Refer to Figure 15-1, which shows a typical primary IV line connecting an IV fluid bag or bottle to the needle or cannula in a vein. The IV **tubing is connected to the IV solution bag** (using sterile technique), and the bag is hung on an IV stand.

Close all roller clamps on the IV tubing before connecting it to the solution bag. This step prevents air bubbles from entering the tubing.

The **drip chamber**, Figure 15-1A, is then squeezed to **half-fill** it with fluid. This level is very important because **IV flow rates are set and monitored by counting the drops falling in this chamber**. If the chamber is too full, the drops cannot be counted. On the other hand, if the outlet at the bottom of the chamber is not completely covered, air can enter the tubing during infusions and, subsequently, the vein and circulatory system. So, the half-full fluid level is extremely important.

The correct fluid level for IV drip chambers is half-full to allow drops to be counted and prevent air from entering the tubing.

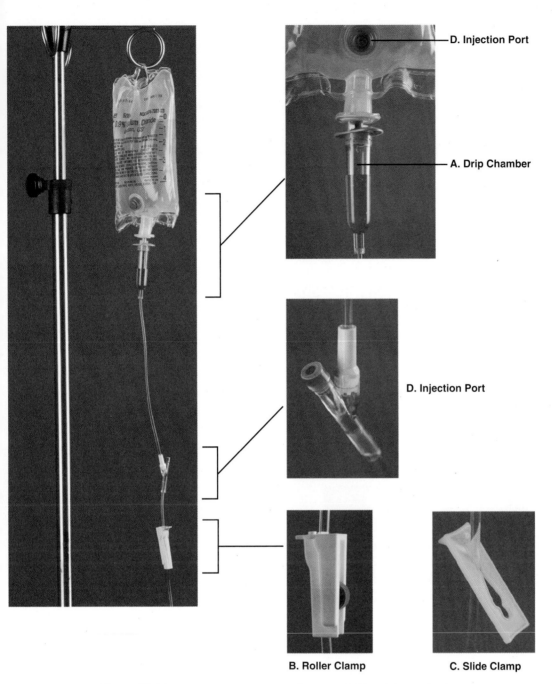

Figure 15-1 | IV tubing and solution bag. Courtesy of Abbott Laboratories.

Next, notice Figure 15-1B, the **roller clamp**. This is adjusted while the drops falling in the drip chamber are counted to **set the flow rate**. It provides an extremely accurate control of rate. A second type of clamp, Figure 15-1C, called a **slide clamp**, is present on all IV tubings. The **slide clamp** can be used to **temporarily stop an IV without disturbing the rate set** on the roller clamp.

Next, notice Figure 15-1D, the **injection port**. Rubber ports are located in several locations on the tubing, typically near the cannula end, drip chamber, and middle of the line, and also on most IV solution bags. **Ports allow injection of medication directly into the line or bag** or the **attachment to the primary line of secondary IV lines** containing compatible IV fluids or medications.

Intravenous fluids run by gravity flow. This necessitates that the IV solution bag be hung **above the patient's heart level** to exert sufficient pressure to infuse. Three feet above heart level is considered an average height.

> The higher an IV bag is hung, the greater the pressure and the faster the IV will infuse.

This pressure differential also means that if the flow rate is adjusted while the patient is lying in bed, it will slow down if he or she sits or stands, and, in fact, it changes slightly with each turn from side to side. For this reason, **monitoring IV flow rate is ongoing,** officially **done every hour,** but routinely checked **after each major position change**.

There are two additional terms relating to primary lines that you must know. If an arm or hand (or, less commonly, leg) vein is used for an infusion, it is referred to as a **peripheral line**. This is to distinguish it from a **central line**, which uses a special catheter whose tip is located centrally **in a deep chest vein**. Central lines may access the chest vein directly through the chest wall, via a neck vein, or through a peripheral vein in the arm or leg.

SECONDARY LINE

Secondary lines attach to the primary line at an injection port. They are used primarily **to infuse medications**, frequently on an intermittent basis; for example, every 6–8 hours. They may also be used to infuse other compatible IV fluids. Secondary lines are commonly referred to as **IV piggybacks**. They are abbreviated **IVPB**. Refer to Figure 15-2, which illustrates a primary and secondary line setup.

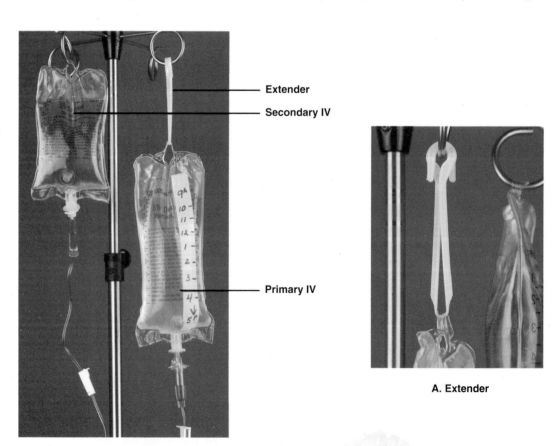

— Extender
— Secondary IV
— Primary IV

A. Extender

Figure 15-2 | Primary and secondary IV setup. Courtesy of Abbott Laboratories.

The IVPB is connected to a port located below the drip chamber on the primary line. Notice that **the IVPB bag is hanging higher than the primary**. This gives it greater pressure and causes it to **infuse first**. Each IVPB set includes a plastic or metal **extender**, in Figure 15-2A, which is used to lower the primary solution bag to obtain this pressure differential. The flow rate for the IVPB is set by a separate roller clamp located on the secondary line. When the IVPB bag has emptied, the primary line will automatically resume its flow. Secondary medication bags are usually much smaller than primary bags. Fifty, 100, 150, 200, and 250 mL bags are frequently used.

Another type of secondary medication setup is provided by Abbott Laboratories **ADD-Vantage System**® (Figure 15-3). In this system, a specially designed IV fluid bag that contains a **medication vial port** is used. The medication vial containing the ordered drug and dosage is inserted into the port, and the drug (frequently in powdered form) is mixed using IV fluid as the diluent, as illustrated in Figure 15-4. The vial contents are then displaced back into the solution bag and thoroughly mixed in the total solution before infusion. The vial remains in the solution bag port throughout the infusion, making it possible to cross-check the vial label for drug and dosage at any time.

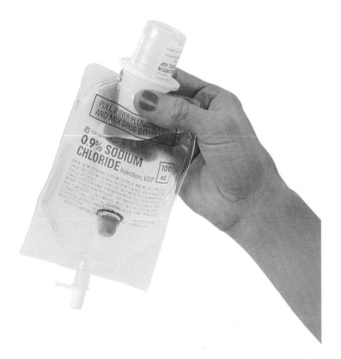

Figure 15-3 | ADD-Vantage System® Courtesy of Abbott
Laboratories.

If a drug is not available in either a prepackaged or ADD-Vantage format, it is often prepared and labeled by the hospital pharmacy. And, finally, an IV medication may be prepared, added to the appropriate IV fluid, thoroughly mixed, labeled and initialed, and administered by the nurse who initiates the infusion.

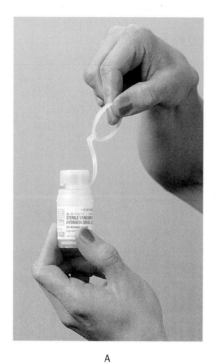

A

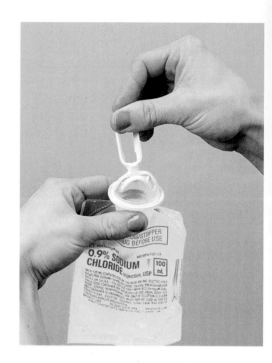

B

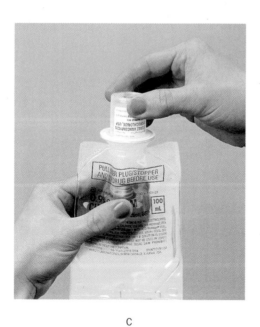

C

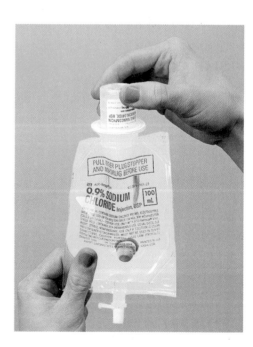

D

Figure 15-4 | ADD-Vantage® System **A,** The ADD-Vantage® medication vial is opened first. **B,** The medication vial port on the IV bag is opened. **C,** The vial top is inserted into the IV bag port and twisted to lock tightly in place. **D,** The vial stopper is removed "inside" the IV bag, and the medication and solution are thoroughly mixed before infusion. Courtesy of Abbott Laboratories.

VOLUME-CONTROLLED BURETTES

For greater accuracy in the measurement of **small-volume** IV medications and fluids, a **calibrated burette chamber** such as the one shown in Figure 15-5 may be used. The total capacity of burettes varies from 100 to 150 mL, calibrated in 1 mL increments. Many burettes are calibrated to deliver very small drops (microdrops), which also contributes to their accuracy. Burettes are most often referred to by their trade names; for example, Buretrols®, Solusets®, or Volutrols®. Burette chambers are most often connected to a secondary solution bag and used as a secondary line, but they can also be primary lines. When medication is ordered, it is injected into the burette through its injection port. The exact amount of IV fluid is then added as a diluent. After thorough mixing, the flow rate is set using a separate clamp on the burette line. Burettes are used extensively in pediatric and intensive care units, where medication dosages and fluid volumes are critical.

INDWELLING INFUSION PORTS/ INTERMITTENT LOCKS

When a continuous IV is not necessary, but intermittent IV medication administration is, an **infusion port adapter** (Figure 15-6) can be attached to an indwelling cannula in a vein. Infusion ports are frequently referred to as **heplocks** or **saline locks (or ports)**. This terminology evolved because the ports must be irrigated with 1–2 mL of sterile saline every 6–8 hours, or with a heparin lock flush solution (100 units/mL) to prevent clotting and blockage. To infuse medication, the port top is cleansed and the medication line is attached. When the infusion is complete, the line is disconnected until the next dosage is due. Ports are also used for **direct injection of medication using a syringe**, which is called an **IV push** or **bolus**.

Heparin anticoagulant therapy will be discussed in detail in a later chapter, where you will learn that heparin is most commonly diluted in large volume intravenous solutions for administration. **The heparin vial dosage strengths available for IV dilution range from 1000 to 50,000 units/mL.** Stop now, and think about the **enormous difference in dosage strengths between heparin flush solutions and intravenous admixture dosages: 10 to 100 units/mL for a flush; 1000 to 50,000 units/mL for IV admixes.**

These large differences in dosage strength demonstrate why **extreme caution is necessary in heparin flush dosage preparation.**

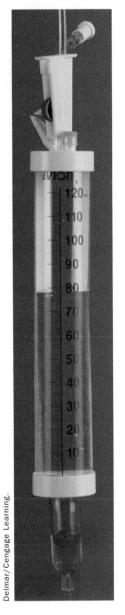

Delmar/Cengage Learning.

Figure 15-5 | A calibrated burette chamber.

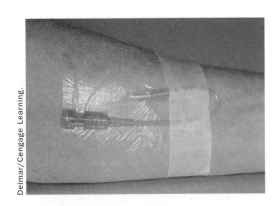

Delmar/Cengage Learning.

Figure 15-6 | An infusion port adapter.

HEPARIN FLUSH DOSAGE ALERT

Heparin flush solutions used to maintain patent (open) indwelling infusion ports come in **two dosage strengths: 10 units/mL and 100 units/mL.** Refer to the Heparin Lock Flush vial label in Figure 15-7 and identify its 10 units/mL strength.

In early 2008 errors in heparin flush dosages became national news when actor Dennis Quaid publicized the near-death of his newborn twins by not one, but two successive errors in flush dosages, which caused the newborns to almost hemorrhage to death.

Thanks to Mr. Quaid, this error was taken all the way to a Congressional hearing to publicize the danger. Similar heparin vial size and label colors were cited as contributing to the errors. But the fact remains that **these errors in dosage were caused by failure to correctly identify label dosage strengths,** not vial size or label color.

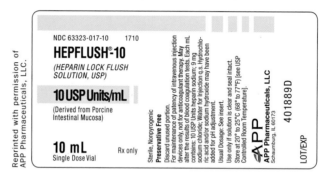

Figure 15-7

 The average heparin flush dosage strength is 10 units and never exceeds 100 units.

Problems 15.1

Answer the questions about IV administration sets as briefly as possible.

1. What is the correct fluid level for an IV drip chamber? _____

2. Which clamp is used to regulate IV flow rate? _____

3. When might a slide clamp be used? _____

4. What is a peripheral line? _____

5. What is a central line? _____

6. What is the common abbreviation for an intravenous piggyback? _____

7. Is the IVPB a primary or secondary line? _____

8. What must the height of a primary solution bag be when a secondary bag is infusing? _____

9. When is a saline lock used?   _____

10. What are the two strengths of heparin
    flush solutions available?   _____

Answers 1. Middle of chamber   **2.** Roller clamp   **3.** Stop the IV temporarily without disturbing
the rate set on the roller clamp   **4.** Arm or leg vein   **5.** IV catheter inserted into a deep chest vein
6. IVPB   **7.** Secondary   **8.** Lower than secondary bag   **9.** For intermittent infusions when a
continuous IV is not necessary   **10.** 10 units/mL and 100 units/mL

VOLUMETRIC PUMPS

Refer now to Figure 15-8 of the Alaris® SE Dual pump. Notice that the IV tubing
with the AccuSlide® flow regulator has been inserted into the channels on the right
and left. The center pumping mechanism maintains the desired flow rates.

All volumetric pumps look similar, and may physically resemble the Alaris SE
pump, but the **functions of different models vary widely**. Some models continue to
pump fluids even if an IV infiltrates, whereas others have a built-in pressure sensor
that will sound an alarm if a resultant increased infusion resistance pressure occurs.
Some models sound an alarm when the solution has completely infused; other
models do not.

Because of the wide variation in pump models and their functions, caution is
mandatory when they are used. It is estimated that a significant number of IV medication errors results from errors in pump programming.

**Hospital or clinical in-service education is required for the use of all
infusion devices.**

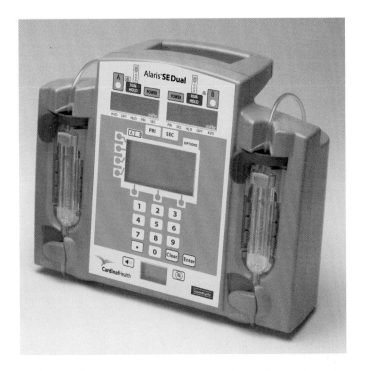

Figure 15-8 | Alaris® SE Dual Pump, with Guardrails. Courtesy of
Cardinal Health, Inc., 2008. All rights reserved.

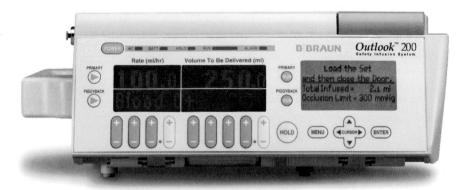

Figure 15-9 | Outlook™ 200 Safety Infusion System. Courtesy of B. Braun Medical, Inc.

Infusion devices are also widely used for IV medication administration, and their precautions in use apply less to the difficulty of the skill than in becoming familiar with the particular infusion model being used. A single hospital or clinic could realistically have a dozen different models in use, and it is an ongoing nursing responsibility to learn how to use each particular model.

 Double-checking of programming is mandatory in the use of infusion devices.

Because errors in infusion device programming are a factor in IV medication errors, it is mandatory that all programming be double-checked. A new generation of sophisticated infusion safety systems has built-in libraries of usual drug dosages, offers customizable drug libraries for facility-specific needs, and is capable of alerting users to programming errors outside hospital-defined parameters. The B. Braun Outlook™ 200 illustrated in Figure 15-9 is one example. Another dose-specific pump is the Alaris System with Guardrails® Suite MX of safety software shown in Figure 15-10, a lightweight, modular platform that integrates infusion, patient monitoring, and clinical best-practice guidelines. As you can clearly see from the photograph, this is an infusion device that requires in-service instruction and certification to use.

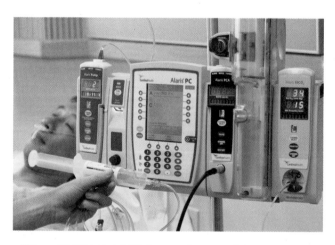

Figure 15-10 | Alaris® PC System. Courtesy of Cardinal Health, 2008. All rights reserved.

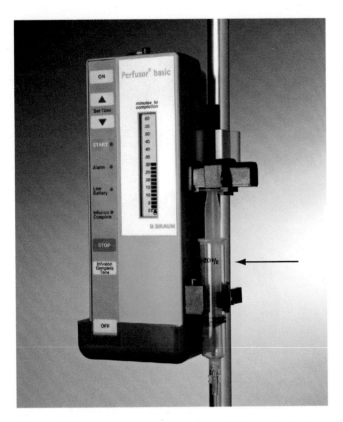

Figure 15-11 | Perfusor® Basic. Courtesy of B. Braun Medical, Inc.

SYRINGE PUMPS

Syringe pumps, as their name implies, are devices that **use a syringe to administer medications or fluids** (Figure 15-11). Syringe pumps are particularly valuable when **drugs that cannot be mixed with other solutions or medications must be administered at a controlled rate over a short period of time**; for example, 5, 10, or 20 minutes. The drug is measured in the syringe, which is inserted into the device, and the medication is infused at the rate set.

PATIENT-CONTROLLED ANALGESIA (PCA) DEVICES

PCA devices allow a patient to **self-administer medication to control pain**. A prefilled syringe or medication bag containing pain medication is inserted into the device (Figure 15-12), and the **dosage and frequency of administration ordered are set**. The patient presses the control button as medication is needed, and the medication is administered and recorded by the PCA.

The device also keeps a record of the number of times a patient **attempts** to use it and thus provides a record of the effectiveness of the dosage prescribed. If a patient's pain is not being relieved, new orders must be obtained and the PCA reset to administer the new dosage.

 All electronic devices must be monitored frequently to be sure they are functioning properly.

Is the IV infusing at the rate that was set? Is the patient who activates a PCA getting relief of pain? If not, is it possible the PCA itself is malfunctioning? Electronic devices have been in use for many years and are relatively trouble-free, but if the desired goal is not being obtained, in the absence of other obvious reasons, **the possibility of malfunction must always be considered**.

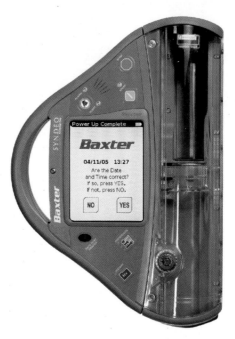

Figure 15-12 | Syndeo PCA (patient-controlled analgesia syringe pump). Courtesy of Baxter Medication Delivery.

Problems 15.2

Answer the questions about infusion devices as briefly as possible.

1. What is the function of a volumetric pump? _____

2. List two major precautions in the use of volumetric pumps. _____

3. When might a syringe pump be used? _____

4. What is a PCA? _____

Answers **1.** To administer IVs at a controlled rate   **2.** Accurate programming; rate and site monitoring
3. To infuse small volumes of drugs that are not compatible with other drugs and/or fluids
4. Patient-controlled analgesia device

INTRODUCTION TO IV FLUIDS

Intravenous fluids are prepared in plastic solution bags or glass bottles in volumes ranging from 50 mL (bags only) to 1000 mL. The 500 and 1000 mL sizes are the most commonly used. The bags and bottles are labeled with the **complete name** of the fluid they contain, and the fine print under the solution name identifies the exact amount of each component of the fluid. **Orders and charting**, however, are done **using abbreviations**.

 In IV fluid abbreviations, D identifies dextrose; W identifies water; S identifies saline; NS identifies normal saline; and numbers identify percentage (%) strengths.

Solutions may be abbreviated in different ways; for example, D5W, 5%D/W, D5%W, or other combinations. But the **initials and percentage have the identical meaning regardless of the way they are abbreviated**. Normal saline solutions are frequently written with the 0.9, or % sign included; for example, D5 0.9NS, or D5 0.9%S. Solutions with different percentages of saline are also available: 0.45%, often written as 1/2 (0.45% is half of 0.9%), and 0.225%, sometimes written as 1/4 (¼ of 0.9) are examples. Some typical orders might be abbreviated D5 1/2S or D5 1/4NS.

Another commonly used solution is **Ringer's lactate**, a balanced electrolyte solution, which is also called Lactated Ringer's Solution. As you would now expect, this solution is abbreviated **RL, LR,** or **RLS**. Electrolytes may also be added to the basic fluids (DW and DS) just discussed. One electrolyte so commonly added that it must be mentioned is **potassium chloride**, which is abbreviated **KCl**. It is measured in milliequivalents **(mEq)**.

Problems 15.3

List the components and percentage strengths of the IV solutions.

1. D10NS   _____

2. D5NS   _____

3. D2.5 1/2S   _____

4. D5 1/4S   _____

5. D20W   _____

6. D5NS 20 mEq KCl   _____

7. D5RL   _____

Answers   1. 10% dextrose in 0.9% saline   **2.** 5% dextrose in normal (0.9%) saline   **3.** 2.5% dextrose in 0.45% saline   **4.** 5% dextrose in 0.225% saline   **5.** 20% dextrose in water   **6.** 5% dextrose in 0.9% saline with 20 mEq potassium chloride   **7.** 5% dextrose in Ringer's lactate solution

PERCENTAGES IN IV FLUIDS

You will recall that **percent means grams of drug per 100 mL of fluid**. This means that a 5% dextrose solution will have 5 g of dextrose in each 100 mL. A 500 mL bag of a 5% solution will contain 5 g × 5, or 25 g of dextrose, whereas 500 mL of a 10% solution contains 10 g × 5, or 50 g of dextrose. The fine print on IV labels always lists the name and amount of all ingredients.

The Ringer's lactate solution in Figure 15-13 illustrates this very well. Take a minute to read the components of this solution.

The point being made here is that **percentages make IV fluids significantly different from each other**. As with drugs, reading labels and making sure the IVs are administered as ordered is critically important.

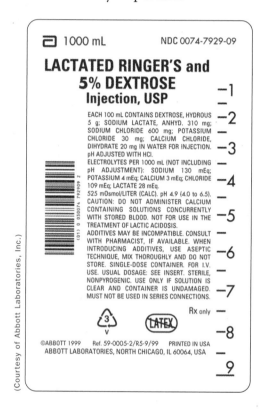

(Courtesy of Abbott Laboratories, Inc.)

Figure 15-13 | IV Solution label: D₅LR.

PARENTERAL NUTRITION

One of the options available for providing nutrition when a patient is unable to eat is to **administer a nutrient solution via a central vein**. This is referred to as parenteral nutrition. The solutions infused are generally of a high caloric content and contain varying percentages of glucose, amino acids, and/or fat emulsions. A number of abbreviations/descriptions are used for parenteral nutrients. Some of the more common are **total parenteral nutrition (TPN), partial parenteral nutrition (PPN), and hyperalimentation (nutrition in excess of maintenance needs)**. There is a noticeable difference in fluids that contain lipids (fat, intralipids) in that they are **opaque-white** in appearance, not unlike nonfat milk. These fluids are normally **infused slowly**, but **not usually over a period of more than 24 hours because they can spoil and support bacterial growth**. All precautions applicable to IVs in general apply equally to parenteral nutrients, with more care necessary for the IV site to prevent infection. Flow rate and infusion time calculations covered in subsequent chapters are also applicable for parenteral nutrition solutions.

Summary

This concludes your introduction to IV therapy. The important points to remember from this chapter are:

- Sterile technique is used to set up all IV solutions, tubings, and devices.

- The correct fluid level for an IV drip chamber is half full.

- Injection ports on an IV line are used to connect secondary lines and to infuse medications.

- A peripheral line refers to an IV infusing in a hand, arm, or leg vein.

- A central line refers to an IV infusing into a deep chest vein.

- IVs flow by gravity pressure, and the higher the solution bag, the faster the IV will infuse.

- The average height for an IV solution bag above the patient's heart level is 3 feet.

- Secondary solution bags must hang higher than the primary bag to infuse first.

- Volume-controlled burettes are used for very exact measurements of IV medications and fluids.

- Intermittent infusion locks or ports are used to infuse IV medications or fluids on an intermittent basis when a continuous IV is not necessary.

- Infusion locks or ports may be irrigated with sterile saline, or heparin flush solutions not to exceed 10–100 units/mL.

- Volumetric pumps are electronic devices that force fluids into a vein under pressure and control infusion rates.

- Syringe pumps are used to infuse medications that cannot be mixed with other fluids or medications.

- Patient-controlled analgesia (PCA) devices allow a patient to self-administer pain medication.

- In IV fluid abbreviations, D identifies dextrose, W identifies water, S identifies saline, NS identifies normal saline, RL or LR identify Ringer's lactated solution, and numbers identify percentage (%) strengths.

Summary Self-Test

You are to assist with some IV procedures. Answer the situational questions concerning these procedures.

1. A patient is admitted and an IV of 1000 mL D5RL is started.
   These initials identify what type of solution?   _____

   This is referred to as what type of IV line?   _____

2. All roller clamps on the IV tubing are closed before connection to the solution bag. Why?   _____

3. The IV is started in the back of the patient's left hand.
   This makes it what type of line?   _____

4. You are asked to check the fluid level in the drip chamber, and you observe that it is correct, which is . . .   _____

5. You are then asked to adjust the flow rate. You will use what type of clamp to do this?   _____

6. It is decided to use an electronic infusion control device to administer this IV. The device used is a . . .   _____

7. An IV antibiotic is ordered for the patient. This is sent from the pharmacy already prepared in a small-volume IV solution bag. The setup used to infuse this medication is referred to as an IV . . .   _____

8. This is abbreviated how?   _____

9. In order for the antibiotic to infuse first, how must it be hung in relation to the original solution bag?   _____

10. Some days later, the patient's IV is to be discontinued, but he is to continue to receive IV antibiotics. What is the site used for this intermittent administration called?   _____

11. The patient had a PCA in use for one day. What do these initials mean?

What does this device control?   _____

Answer these as briefly as possible.

12. A small-volume IV medication is to be diluted in 20 mL and infused. This can be most accurately measured using a _____.

13. These devices are calibrated in _____ increments.

14. When an IV medication is injected directly into the vein via a port, it is called an IV _____ or _____.

15. What heparin dosage strengths are used for IV port flush?   _____

16. Ports may be irrigated with _____ mL of _____ to prevent blockage every _____ hours.

17. In IV fluid abbreviations, D5NS identifies what IV fluid?   _____

Answers

1. 5% dextrose in Ringer's lactate; primary
2. To prevent air from entering the tubing
3. Peripheral
4. Half full
5. Roller
6. Volumetric pump
7. Piggyback
8. IVPB
9. Higher
10. Intermittent infusion port; saline or heparin lock
11. Patient-controlled analgesia; administration of pain medication
12. Calibrated burette
13. 1 mL
14. Push or bolus
15. 10 units/mL or 100 units/mL
16. 1–2; normal saline; 6–8
17. 5% dextrose in normal saline

IV FLOW RATE CALCULATION

16

Objectives

The learner will:

1. identify the calibrations in gtt/mL on IV administration sets.

2. calculate flow rates using dimensional analysis.

3. calculate flow rates using the formula and division factor methods.

4. recalculate flow rates to correct off-schedule infusions.

This chapter presents three ways to calculate IV flow rates using dimensional analysis, the formula method, and the division factor method.

Intravenous fluids are ordered on the basis of **mL/hr** to be administered; for example, 125 mL/hr. With the widespread use of electronic infusion devices that can be **set to deliver a mL/hr rate**, simply setting the rate ordered on the device and making sure it is working properly is all that is required for many infusions.

The most common flow rate calculation is necessary **when an infusion device is not being used.** It involves **converting a mL/hr order to the gtt/min rate necessary to infuse it**; for example, **1000 mL to infuse at 125 mL/hr** or **3000 mL/24 hr**.

IV TUBING CALIBRATION

The size of IV drops is regulated by the type of IV set being used, which is **calibrated in number of gtt/mL.** Unfortunately, not all sets (or their drop size) are the same. Each clinical facility uses at least two sizes of infusion sets: a standard **macrodrip set calibrated at 10, 15, or 20 gtt/mL** which is used for routine adult IV administrations, and a **microdrip set calibrated at 60 gtt/mL** which is used when more exact measurements are needed; for example, to infuse medications or in critical care and pediatric infusions. Figure 16-1 gives a graphic representation of the various drop/gtt sizes.

 IV administration sets are calibrated in gtt/mL.

The **gtt/mL calibration of each IV infusion set is clearly printed on each package**, and the first step in calculating flow rates is to identify the gtt/mL calibration of the set to be used for an infusion.

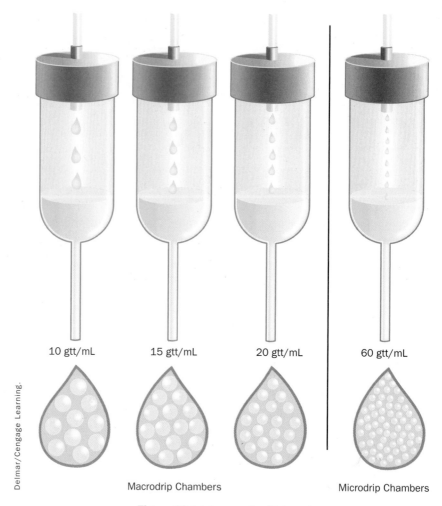

Figure 16-1 | Comparative IV drop sizes.

Problems 16.1

Identify the calibration in gtt/mL for each IV infusion set.

1. Figure 16-2 _____

2. Figure 16-3 _____

3. Figure 16-4 _____

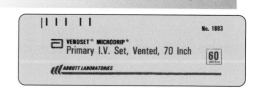

Figure 16-2 | Courtesy of Abbott Laboratories.

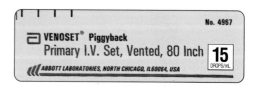

Figure 16-3 | Courtesy of Abbott Laboratories.

Answers **1.** 60 gtt/mL **2.** 15 gtt/mL **3.** 10 gtt/mL

2C5419s

Baxter-Travenol

Vented Basic Set

10 drops/mL

10

Figure 16-4 | Courtesy of Baxter Healthcare.

CALCULATING gtt/min FLOW RATES FROM mL/hr ORDERED

The flow rate in **gtt/min** is calculated from the **calibration of the IV set being used**, either 10, 15, 20, or 60 gtt/mL, and the **mL/hr ordered**. You will immediately notice a difference from the previous DA calculations you have learned because **this calculation includes two values: gtt and min**. However, the DA calculation steps are identical.

EXAMPLE 1   Calculate a **gtt/min** flow rate to infuse **125 mL/hr** using a set calibrated at **10 gtt/mL**.

- Enter the **gtt/min** to be calculated as a **common fraction** followed by an equal sign.

$$\frac{gtt}{min} =$$

- **Begin ratio entries as if you were calculating only the gtt numerator.** Locate the ratio containing gtt—the 10 gtt/mL set calibration. Enter 10 gtt as the numerator to match the gtt numerator being calculated; 1 mL becomes the denominator.

$$\frac{gtt}{min} = \frac{10\ gtt}{1\ mL}$$

- Match the mL denominator with the 125 mL of the 125 mL/hr ordered; 1 hr becomes the denominator.

$$\frac{gtt}{min} = \frac{10\ gtt}{1\ mL} \times \frac{125\ mL}{1\ hr}$$

- **Enter a 1 hr equals 60 min conversion ratio,** with 1 hr as the numerator and 60 min as the denominator. Notice that **the min being calculated falls automatically into place** as the final denominator to complete the equation.

$$\frac{gtt}{min} = \frac{10\ gtt}{1\ mL} \times \frac{125\ mL}{1\ hr} \times \frac{1\ hr}{60\ min}$$

- Cancel the mL, mL and hr, and hr denominator/numerators to check for correct ratio entry. Do the math.

$$\frac{gtt}{min} = \frac{10\ gtt}{1\ \cancel{mL}} \times \frac{125\ \cancel{mL}}{1\ \cancel{hr}} \times \frac{1\ \cancel{hr}}{60\ min} = 20.8 = \textbf{21 gtt/min}$$

To infuse 125 mL/hr using a 10 gtt/mL infusion set, the flow rate is 21 gtt/min.

   Flow rates are rounded to the nearest whole gtt.

EXAMPLE 2   A **20 gtt/mL** set is used to infuse **90 mL/hr**. Calculate the **gtt/min** flow rate.

- Enter the gtt/min to be calculated followed by an equal sign.

$$\frac{gtt}{min} =$$

- Enter the 20 gtt/mL infusion set ratio with 20 gtt to match the gtt numerator being calculated; 1 mL becomes the denominator.

$$\frac{gtt}{min} = \frac{20 \ gtt}{1 \ mL}$$

- Match the mL denominator with the 90 mL of the mL/hr ordered; 1 hr is the new denominator.

$$\frac{gtt}{min} = \frac{20 \ gtt}{1 \ mL} \times \frac{90 \ mL}{1 \ hr}$$

- Enter a 1 hr equals 60 min conversion ratio, with 1 hr as the numerator and 60 min as the denominator, to complete the equation.

$$\frac{gtt}{min} = \frac{20 \ gtt}{1 \ mL} \times \frac{90 \ mL}{1 \ hr} \times \frac{1 \ hr}{60 \ min}$$

- Cancel the mL, mL and hr, and hr denominator/numerators to check for correct ratio entry. Do the math.

$$\frac{gtt}{min} = \frac{20 \ gtt}{1 \ \cancel{mL}} \times \frac{90 \ \cancel{mL}}{1 \ \cancel{hr}} \times \frac{1 \ \cancel{hr}}{60 \ min} = \textbf{30 gtt/min}$$

To infuse 90 mL/hr using a set calibrated at 20 gtt/mL, the rate is 30 gtt/min.

EXAMPLE 3   Calculate the **gtt/min** rate to infuse **2500 mL** in **24 hr** using a **15 gtt/mL** infusion set.

- Enter the gtt/min to be calculated followed by an equal sign.

$$\frac{gtt}{min} =$$

- Enter the 15 gtt/mL infusion set ratio with 15 gtt to match the gtt numerator being calculated; 1 mL becomes the denominator.

$$\frac{gtt}{min} = \frac{15 \ gtt}{1 \ mL}$$

- Enter the 2500 mL/24 hr ordered with 2500 mL as the numerator to match the previous mL denominator. Enter 24 hr as the new denominator.

$$\frac{gtt}{min} = \frac{15 \ gtt}{1 \ mL} \times \frac{2500 \ mL}{24 \ hr}$$

- Enter a 1 hr equals 60 min conversion ratio, with 1 hr as the numerator and 60 min as the denominator, to complete the equation.

$$\frac{gtt}{min} = \frac{15\ gtt}{1\ mL} \times \frac{2500\ mL}{24\ hr} \times \frac{1\ hr}{60\ min}$$

- Cancel the mL, mL and hr, and hr denominator/numerators to check for correct ratio entry. Do the math.

$$\frac{gtt}{min} = \frac{15\ gtt}{1\ \cancel{mL}} \times \frac{2500\ \cancel{mL}}{24\ \cancel{hr}} \times \frac{1\ \cancel{hr}}{60\ min} = 26.04 = \textbf{26 gtt/min}$$

To infuse 2500 mL in 24 hr using a 15 gtt/mL calibrated infusion set, the rate is 26 gtt/min.

EXAMPLE 4   Calculate the **gtt/min** rate to infuse **2000 mL** in **10 hr** using a **10 gtt/mL** IV infusion set.

- Enter the gtt/min to be calculated followed by an equal sign.

$$\frac{gtt}{min} =$$

- Enter the 10 gtt/mL infusion set ratio with 10 gtt as the numerator to match the gtt numerator being calculated; 1 mL becomes the denominator.

$$\frac{gtt}{min} = \frac{10\ gtt}{1\ mL}$$

- Enter the 2000 mL in 10 hr ordered with 2000 mL as the numerator to match the previous mL denominator; 10 hr is the next denominator to be matched.

$$\frac{gtt}{min} = \frac{10\ gtt}{1\ mL} \times \frac{2000\ mL}{10\ hr}$$

- Enter a 1 hr equals 60 min conversion ratio, with 1 hr as the numerator and 60 min as the denominator, to complete the equation.

$$\frac{gtt}{min} = \frac{10\ gtt}{1\ mL} \times \frac{2000\ mL}{10\ hr} \times \frac{1\ hr}{60\ min}$$

- Cancel the mL, mL and hr, and hr denominator/numerators to check for correct ratio entry. Do the math.

$$\frac{gtt}{min} = \frac{10\ gtt}{1\ \cancel{mL}} \times \frac{2000\ \cancel{mL}}{10\ \cancel{hr}} \times \frac{1\ \cancel{hr}}{60\ min} = 33.3 = \textbf{33 gtt/min}$$

To infuse 2000 mL in 10 hr using a 10 gtt/mL calibrated infusion set, the rate is 33 gtt/min.

Problems 16.2

Calculate gtt/min flow rates. Round to the nearest whole gtt.

1. An IV of 2000 mL is to infuse in 12 hr using a 10 gtt/mL set. _____

2. 3500 mL are ordered to infuse in 24 hr using a set calibrated at 20 gtt/mL. _____

3. Infuse 500 mL in 3 hr using a 15 gtt/mL set. _____

4. A volume of 1500 mL is to infuse in 5 hr using a 15 gtt/mL set. _____

5. 1750 mL are ordered to infuse in 9 hr using a 20 gtt/mL set. _____

6. An IV of 2500 mL is to infuse in 18 hr on a set calibrated at 10 gtt/mL. _____

7. A 3000 mL volume is to infuse in 24 hr on a set calibrated at 20 gtt/mL. _____

8. A volume of 2750 mL is to infuse in 22 hr on a 15 gtt/mL set. _____

9. An IV of 750 mL is ordered to infuse in 8 hr on a 10 gtt/mL set. _____

10. A volume of 1250 mL is to infuse in 12 hr using a 15 gtt/mL set. _____

Answers   1. 28 gtt/min   **2.** 49 gtt/min   **3.** 42 gtt/min   **4.** 75 gtt/min   **5.** 65 gtt/min   **6.** 23 gtt/min
7. 42 gtt/min   **8.** 31 gtt/min   **9.** 16 gtt/min   **10.** 26 gtt/min

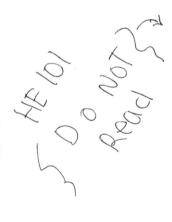

FORMULA AND DIVISION FACTOR METHODS OF FLOW RATE CALCULATION

The **formula** and **division factor** methods are intrinsically related because **the division factor is derived from the formula method**. Let's start by looking at the formula method.

The formula method has a limitation in that it can **only be used if the flow rate is expressed as mL/hr (60 min) or less**; for example, 110 mL/60 min or 125 mL/60 min. It is especially suitable for small-volume infusions to be completed in less than 60 min; for example, 30 mL in 20 min.

$$\text{Flow Rate} = \frac{\text{mL/hr Volume} \times \text{Set Calibration}}{\text{Time (60 min or less)}}$$

EXAMPLE 1 An IV of 500 mL is ordered to infuse at **125 mL/hr**. Calculate the **gtt/min** rate for a set calibrated at **10 gtt/mL**.

- **Convert the hr rate to 60 min.**

$$\frac{125(\text{mL}) \times 10(\text{gtt/mL})}{60(\text{min})}$$

- **Calculate the gtt/min rate.**

$$\frac{125 \times 10}{60} = 20.8 = \textbf{21 gtt/min}$$

EXAMPLE 2 Administer an IV medication of **100 mL** in **40 min** using a set calibrated at **15 gtt/mL**.

$$\frac{100 \text{ mL} \times 15 \text{ gtt/mL}}{40 \text{ min}} = 37.5 = \textbf{38 gtt/min}$$

EXAMPLE 3 A **75 mL** volume of IV medication is ordered to infuse in **45 min**. The set is calibrated at **20 gtt/mL**.

$$\frac{75 \text{ mL} \times 20 \text{ gtt/mL}}{45 \text{ min}} = 33.3 = \textbf{33 gtt/min}$$

Problems 16.3

Calculate the flow rate in gtt/min to the nearest whole drop using the formula method.

1. Administer an IV of 110 mL/hr using a set calibrated at 20 gtt/mL. _____

2. A 500 mL IV solution is ordered to infuse at 200 mL/hr using a set calibrated at 15 gtt/mL. _____

3. A volume of 80 mL is to be infused in 20 min using a 10 gtt/mL set. _____

4. An IV of 1000 mL is ordered to infuse at 150 mL/hr using a 10 gtt/mL calibrated set. _____

5. An IV rate of 90 mL/hr is ordered using a 15 gtt/mL calibrated set. _____

6. An IV of 500 mL is to infuse at 120 mL/hr using a 20 gtt/mL calibrated set. _____

7. A total of 90 mL is to infuse at 100 mL/hr using a 20 gtt/mL set. _____

8. A 15 gtt/mL set is used to infuse 120 mL at 80 mL/hr. _____

9. A rate of 60 mL/hr is ordered for a volume of 250 mL using a 10 gtt/mL set. _____

10. A medication volume of 50 mL is to infuse at 20 mL/hr using a 20 gtt/mL set. _____

Answers 1. 37 gtt/min **2.** 50 gtt/min **3.** 40 gtt/min **4.** 25 gtt/min **5.** 23 gtt/min
6. 40 gtt/min **7.** 33 gtt/min **8.** 20 gtt/min **9.** 10 gtt/min **10.** 7 gtt/min

When an IV is ordered to infuse in **more than 1 hour**, the formula method can still be used. However, it is necessary to add a preliminary step and determine the **mL/hr** the ordered volume will represent.

EXAMPLE 1   Calculate the gtt/min flow rate for an IV of **1000 mL** to infuse in **8 hr** on a set calibrated at **20 gtt/mL**.

- **Convert 1000 mL/8 hr to mL/hr.**

  1000 mL/8 hr = 1000 ÷ 8 = **125 mL/hr (60 min)**

- **Calculate the gtt/min flow rate.**

  $$\frac{125\ (\text{mL}) \times 20\,(\text{gtt/mL})}{60\ (\text{min})} = 41.6 = \textbf{42 gtt/min}$$

EXAMPLE 2   Calculate the gtt/min flow rate for a volume of **2500 mL** to infuse in **24 hr** on a set calibrated at **10 gtt/mL**.

- **Convert 2500 mL/24 hr to mL/hr.**

  2500 mL/24 hr = 2500 ÷ 24 = **104 mL/hr (60 min)**

- **Calculate the gtt/min flow rate.**

  $$\frac{104\ \text{mL} \times 10\ \text{gtt/mL}}{60\ \text{min}} = 17.3 = \textbf{17 gtt/min}$$

EXAMPLE 3   An IV of **1200 mL** is to infuse in **16 hr** on a set calibrated at **15 gtt/mL**.

1200 mL/16 hr = 1200 ÷ 16 = **75 mL/hr (60 min)**

$$\frac{75\ \text{mL} \times 15\ \text{gtt/mL}}{60\ \text{min}} = 18.7 = \textbf{19 gtt/min}$$

Problems 16.4

Calculate the gtt/min flow rate using the formula method.

1. A volume of 2000 mL to infuse in 24 hr on a set calibrated at 15 gtt/mL.   _____

2. A volume of 300 mL to infuse in 6 hr on a 60 gtt/mL microdrip set.   _____

3. A volume of 500 mL to infuse in 4 hr on a 15 gtt/mL calibrated set.   _____

4. A 10 hr infusion of 1200 mL using a 20 gtt/mL set.   _____

5. An infusion of 500 mL in 5 hr on a set calibrated at 10 gtt/mL.   _____

6. A 2000 mL volume to infuse in 18 hr using a
   20 gtt/mL set.   _____

7. A 10 gtt/mL set to infuse 400 mL in 4 hr.   _____

8. An 8 hr infusion of 1500 mL to use a set calibrated
   at 15 gtt/mL.   _____

9. A volume of 250 mL to infuse in 2 hr using a
   20 gtt/mL set.   _____

10. A 5 hr infusion of 750 mL using a 10 gtt/mL set. _____

Answers 1. 21 gtt/min   **2.** 50 gtt/min   **3.** 31 gtt/min   **4.** 40 gtt/min   **5.** 17 gtt/min   **6.** 37 gtt/min
7. 17 gtt/min   **8.** 47 gtt/min   **9.** 42 gtt/min   **10.** 25 gtt/min

DIVISION FACTOR METHOD

The **division factor** is derived from the formula method, and it is invaluable for
use in clinical facilities where **all the macrodrip infusion sets have the same
calibration**—either 10, 15, or 20 gtt/mL. Once again, **this method can only be
used if the rate is expressed in mL/hr (60 min)**. Let's start by looking at how the
division factor is obtained.

EXAMPLE   Administer an IV at **125 mL/hr**. The set calibration is **10 gtt/mL**.
Calculate the gtt/min rate. Express the hr rate as 60 min.

$$\frac{125(\text{mL}) \times \overset{1}{\cancel{10}}(\text{gtt/mL})}{\underset{6}{\cancel{60}}(\text{min})} = 20.8 = \textbf{21 gtt/min}$$

Look at the completed equation, and notice that because the time is restricted to
60 min, **the set calibration (10) will be divided into 60 (min) to obtain a constant
number (6). This constant (6) is the division factor for a 10 gtt/mL calibrated set.**

 The division factor can be obtained for any IV set by dividing
60 by the calibration of the set.

Problems 16.5

Determine the division factor for these IV sets.

1. 20 gtt/mL   _____

2. 15 gtt/mL   _____

3. 60 gtt/mL   _____

4. 10 gtt/mL   _____

Answers   1. 3   **2.** 4   **3.** 1   **4.** 6

Once the division factor is known, **the gtt/min rate can be calculated in one step by dividing the mL/hr rate by the division factor**. Look again at the example.

$$\frac{125(\text{mL}) \times \overset{1}{\cancel{10}}(\text{gtt/mL})}{\underset{6}{\cancel{60}}(\text{min})} = 20.8 = \textbf{21 gtt/min}$$

or $125(\text{mL/hr}) \div \textbf{6} = 20.8 = \textbf{21 gtt/min}$

The 125 mL/hr flow rate divided by the division factor 6 gives the same 21 gtt/min rate.

The gtt/min flow rate can be calculated for mL/hr IV orders in one step by dividing the mL/hr to be infused by the division factor of the administration set.

EXAMPLE 1   Infuse an IV at **100 mL/hr** using a set calibrated at **10 gtt/mL**.

Determine the division factor: $60 \div 10 = \textbf{6}$

Calculate the flow rate: $100 \text{ mL} \div 6 = 16.6 = \textbf{17 gtt/min}$

EXAMPLE 2   Infuse an IV at **125 mL/hr** using a set calibrated at **15 gtt/mL**.

$60 \div 15 = \textbf{4}$ $\qquad\qquad$ $125 \text{ mL} \div 4 = 31.2 = \textbf{31 gtt/min}$

EXAMPLE 3   A set calibrated at **20 gtt/mL** is used to infuse **90 mL per hr**.

$60 \div 20 = \textbf{3}$ $\qquad\qquad$ $90 \text{ mL} \div 3 = \textbf{30 gtt/min}$

Problems 16.6

Calculate the flow rates in gtt/min using the division factor method.

1. A rate of 110 mL/hr via a set calibrated at 20 gtt/mL.   _____
2. A set is calibrated at 15 gtt/mL. Infuse at 130 mL/hr.   _____
3. To infuse 150 mL/hr using a 10 gtt/mL set.   _____
4. A set calibrated at 20 gtt/mL to infuse 45 mL/hr.   _____
5. A 75 mL/hr volume with a set calibrated at 15 gtt/mL.   _____
6. A rate of 130 mL/hr using a 10 gtt/mL set.   _____
7. A 200 mL rate using a 15 gtt/mL set.   _____
8. A rate of 120 mL/hr using a 10 gtt/mL set.   _____
9. A 100 mL/hr rate using a 20 gtt/mL set.   _____
10. A rate of 125 mL/hr using a 15 gtt/mL set.   _____

Answers **1.** 37 gtt/min **2.** 33 gtt/min **3.** 25 gtt/min **4.** 15 gtt/min **5.** 19 gtt/min **6.** 22 gtt/min **7.** 50 gtt/min **8.** 20 gtt/min **9.** 33 gtt/min **10.** 31 gtt/min

All the preceding examples and problems using the division factor were for **macrodrip** sets. Let's now look at what happens when a **microdrip** set calibrated at **60 gtt/mL** is used.

> **EXAMPLE**   Infuse at **50 mL/hr** using a **60 gtt/mL** microdrip.
>
> $$60 \div 60 = 1 \qquad\qquad 50 \text{ mL} \div 1 = \textbf{50 gtt/min}$$

Because the set calibration is 60 and the division factor is based on 60 min (1 hr), the division factor is 1. So, **for microdrip sets, the gtt/min flow rate will be identical to the mL/hr ordered**.

 When a 60 gtt/mL microdrip set is used, the flow rate in gtt/min is identical to the volume in mL/hr to be infused.

Problems 16.7

Calculate gtt/min rates for a microdrip.

1. 120 mL/hr _____
2. 90 mL/hr _____
3. 100 mL/hr _____
4. 75 mL/hr _____
5. 80 mL/hr _____

6. 110 mL/hr _____
7. 60 mL/hr _____
8. 45 mL/hr _____
9. 70 mL/hr _____
10. 130 mL/hr _____

Answers 1. 120 gtt/min **2.** 90 gtt/min **3.** 100 gtt/min **4.** 75 gtt/min **5.** 80 gtt/min
6. 110 gtt/min **7.** 60 gtt/min **8.** 45 gtt/min **9.** 70 gtt/min **10.** 130 gtt/min

The division factor can also be used to calculate the flow rate of **any volume that can be expressed in mL/hr**. Larger volumes can be divided, and smaller volumes can be multiplied and expressed in mL/hr. This does require the conversion step you used earlier.

> **EXAMPLE 1** $2400 \text{ mL}/24 \text{ hr} = 2400 \div 24 = \textbf{100 mL/hr}$

> **EXAMPLE 2** $1800 \text{ mL}/8 \text{ hr} = 1800 \div 8 = \textbf{225 mL/hr}$

> **EXAMPLE 3** $10 \text{ mL}/30 \text{ min} = 10 \times 2 (2 \times 30 \text{ min}) = \textbf{20 mL/hr}$

> **EXAMPLE 4** $15 \text{ mL}/20 \text{ min} = 15 \times 3 (3 \times 20 \text{ min}) = \textbf{45 mL/hr}$

REGULATING FLOW RATE

Manual flow rates are regulated by **counting the number of drops falling in the drip chamber**. The standard procedure for counting is to hold a watch next to the drip chamber and actually **count the number of drops falling**. The roller clamp is adjusted during the count until the required rate has been set. A 15 sec count is most commonly used because there is less chance of attention wandering during the count. This means that the ordered gtt/min (60 sec) rate must be divided by 4 to obtain the 15 sec drip count (60 sec ÷ 4 = 15 sec).

EXAMPLE 1   An IV is to run at a rate of **60 gtt/min**. What will the 15 sec count be?

60 gtt/min ÷ 4 = **15 gtt**

Adjust the rate to 15 gtt/15 sec.

EXAMPLE 2   A 70 **gtt/min** IV rate is ordered. What will the 15 sec count be?

70 gtt/min ÷ 4 = 17.5 = **18 gtt**

Adjust the rate to 18 gtt/15 sec.

EXAMPLE 3   Adjust an IV to a rate of **50 gtt/min** using a 15 sec count.

50 gtt/min ÷ 4 = **13 gtt**

Adjust the rate to 13 gtt/15 sec.

Problems 16.8

Answer the questions about 15 sec drip rates.

1. The 15 second count of an IV flow rate is 7 gtt. A 29 gtt/min rate is required. Is this rate correct? _____

2. You are to regulate a newly started IV to deliver 67 gtt/min. Using a 15 second count, how would you set the flow rate? _____

3. An IV is to run at 48 gtt/min. What must the 15 second drip rate be? _____

4. How many gtt will you count in 15 sec if the rate is 55 gtt/min? _____

5. An IV is to run at 84 gtt/min. What will the 15 sec rate be? _____

6. What must the 15 sec count be to infuse 80 gtt/min? _____

7. A 110 gtt/min rate is ordered. What must the 15 sec count be? _____

8. A 100 gtt/min rate is ordered. What must the 15 sec count be? _____

9. A rate of 90 gtt/min is ordered. Is a count of 15 gtt in
   15 sec correct? _____

10. An IV is infusing at a rate of 30 gtt in 15 sec.
    A rate of 120 gtt/min was ordered. Is this rate correct? _____

Answers **1.** Yes **2.** 17 gtt/15 sec **3.** 12 gtt/15 sec **4.** 14 gtt/15 sec **5.** 21 gtt/15 sec
6. 20 gtt/15 sec **7.** 28 gtt/15 sec **8.** 25 gtt/15 sec **9.** No, too slow **10.** Yes

Individual clinical facilities and/or states/provinces may require a 30 or 60 sec
(1 min) count. When a 60 sec count is required, particular care must be taken not to
let your attention wander during the count, which can easily happen in this longer
time frame. A 60 sec count will require a 1 min count, whereas a 30 sec count will
require the gtt/min rate to be divided by 2 (60 sec ÷ 2 = 30 sec).

EXAMPLE 1   An IV is to be infused at 56 gtt/min. What is the 30 sec rate?

56 gtt/min ÷ 2 = 28 gtt

Adjust the rate to 28 gtt/30 sec.

EXAMPLE 2   A rate of 72 gtt/min has been ordered. What will the 30 sec
count be?

72 gtt/min ÷ 2 = 36 gtt

Adjust the rate to 36 gtt/30 sec.

Problems 16.9

Calculate a 30 sec flow rate count.

1. An IV to be run at a rate of 48 gtt/min.   _____
2. An IV ordered to infuse at 52 gtt/min.   _____
3. An IV to infuse at 120 gtt/min.   _____
4. An infusion rate of 90 gtt/min.   _____
5. An IV to infuse at 100 gtt/min.   _____

Answers **1.** 24 gtt/30 sec **2.** 26 gtt/30 sec **3.** 60 gtt/30 sec **4.** 45 gtt/30 sec **5.** 50 gtt/30 sec

CORRECTING OFF-SCHEDULE RATES

Because positional changes can alter the rate slightly, IVs occasionally infuse ahead
of or behind schedule. When this occurs, the usual procedure is to **recalculate the
flow rate using the volume and time remaining** and to **adjust the rate accordingly**. However, each situation must be individually evaluated, especially if the
discrepancy is large. **If too much fluid has infused, immediately assess the individual's response** to the increased intake and take appropriate action. **If too little
fluid has infused**, it will be necessary to **assess the individual's ability to tolerate
an increased rate** because many medications and fluids have restrictions on the

rate of administration. Both of these factors must be considered before rates can be increased to "catch up." In addition, **most clinical facilities will have specific policies to cover over- or under infusion due to altered flow rates, and you will be responsible for knowing these.**

The following are some examples of how the rate can be recalculated. Because IVs are usually checked hourly, the focus will first be on recalculation using exact hours. Some recalculations have also been included using fractions of hours rounded to the nearest quarter hour: 15 min = 0.25 hr, 30 min = 0.5 hr, and 45 min = 0.75 hr. These equivalents are close enough for uncomplicated infusions because the exact time of completion is not totally predictable. IVs needing exact infusion would be monitored by electronic infusion devices.

EXAMPLE 1

An IV of **1000 mL** was ordered to infuse over **10 hr** at a rate of **25 gtt/min**. The set calibration is **15 gtt/mL**. After **5 hr**, a total of 650 mL have infused instead of the **500 mL** ordered. Recalculate the new gtt/min flow rate to complete the infusion on schedule.

Time remaining   10 hr − 5 hr = **5 hr**

Volume remaining   1000 mL − 650 mL = **350 mL**

350 mL ÷ 5 hr = **70 mL/hr**

Set calibration is **15 gtt/mL**.

70 ÷ 4(division factor) = 17.5 = **18 gtt/min**

Slow the rate from 25 gtt/min to 18 gtt/min.

EXAMPLE 2

An IV of **800 mL** was to infuse over **8 hr** at **20 gtt/min**. After **4 hr 15 min** only **300 mL** have infused. Recalculate the **gtt/min** rate to complete on schedule. The set calibration is **15 gtt/mL**.

Time remaining   8 hr − 4.25 hr = **3.75 hr**

Volume remaining   800 mL − 300 mL = **500 mL**

500 mL ÷ 3.75 hr = 133.3 = **133 mL/hr**

Set calibration is **15 gtt/mL**.

133 ÷ 4(division factor) = 33.2 = **33 gtt/min**

Increase the rate to 33 gtt/min.

EXAMPLE 3

An IV of **500 mL** is infusing at **28 gtt/min**. It was to complete in **3 hr**, but after **1½ hr**, only **175 mL** have infused. Recalculate the **gtt/min** rate to complete the infusion on schedule. Set calibration is **10 gtt/mL**.

Time remaining   3 hr − 1.5 hr = **1.5 hr**

Volume remaining   500 mL − 175 mL = **325 mL**

325 mL ÷ 1.5 hr = 216.6 = **217 mL/hr**

Set calibration is **10 gtt/mL**.

$217 \div 6(\text{division factor}) = 36.1 = \textbf{36 gtt/min}$

Increase the rate to 36 gtt/min.

EXAMPLE 4   A volume of **250 mL** was to infuse **56 gtt/min** in **1½ hr** using a set calibrated at **20 gtt/mL**. After **30 min**, **175 mL** have infused. Recalculate the flow rate.

Time remaining   1.5 hr $-$ 30 min $= \textbf{1 hr}$

Volume remaining   250 mL $-$ 175 mL $= \textbf{75 mL}$

Set calibration is **20 gtt/mL**.

$75 \div 3(\text{division factor}) = \textbf{25 gtt/min}$

Decrease the rate to 25 gtt/min.

Problems 16.10

Recalculate flow rates for infusions to complete on schedule.

1. An IV of 500 mL was ordered to infuse in 3 hr using a 15 gtt/mL set. With 1½ hr remaining, you discover that only 150 mL is left in the bag. At what rate will you need to reset the flow? _____

2. An IV of 1000 mL was scheduled to run in 12 hr. After 4 hr, only 220 mL have infused. The set calibration is 20 gtt/mL. Recalculate the rate for the remaining solution. _____

3. An IV of 1000 mL was ordered to infuse in 8 hr. With 3 hr of infusion time left, you discover that 600 mL have infused. The set delivers 20 gtt/mL. Recalculate the drip rate, and indicate how many drops you will count in 15 sec to set the new rate. _____ _____

4. An IV of 750 mL was ordered to run in 6 hr with a set calibrated at 10 gtt/mL. After 2 hr, you notice that 300 mL have infused. Recalculate the flow rate, and indicate how many drops you will count in 15 sec to reset the rate. _____ _____

5. An IV of 800 mL was started at 9 am to infuse in 4 hr. At 10 am 150 mL have infused. The set is calibrated at 15 gtt/mL. Recalculate the flow rate in gtt/min. _____

6. An IV of 600 mL was to infuse in 5 hr. After 2 hr, 400 mL have infused. Recalculate the gtt/min rate to complete on time. A 20 gtt/mL set is being used. _____

7. A volume of 250 mL was to infuse in 2 hr. With 1 hr left, 70 mL have infused. Calculate a new gtt/min rate to complete on time using a 15 gtt/mL set. _____

8. An infiltrated IV is restarted with a volume of 420 mL to complete in 3 hr. Calculate the gtt/min rate for a 20 gtt/mL set. What will the new 30 sec count be? _____   _____

9. After 1 hr 30 min, 350 mL of a 1000 mL IV has infused. It was ordered to complete in 4 hr using a set calibrated at 15 gtt/mL. Calculate the gtt/min rate to complete on time. _____

10. A total of 300 mL of an ordered 1000 mL in 10 hr infusion has completed in 4.5 hr. The set calibration is 15 gtt/mL. What gtt/min rate is necessary to complete on time? Calculate the 15 sec count to deliver this rate. _____   _____

Answers   1. 25 gtt/min   **2.** 33 gtt/min   **3.** 44 gtt/min; 11 gtt/15 sec   **4.** 19 gtt/min; 4–5 gtt/15 sec   **5.** 54 gtt/min   **6.** 22 gtt/min   **7.** 45 gtt/min   **8.** 47 gtt/min; 23–24 gtt/30 sec   **9.** 65 gtt/min   **10.** 32 gtt/min; 8 gtt/15 sec

Summary

This concludes the chapter on IV flow rate calculation and monitoring. The important points to remember from this chapter are:

- IVs are ordered as mL/hr to be administered.

- Manual flow rates are counted in gtt/min.

- IV tubings are calibrated in gtt/mL.

- Macrodrip IV sets have a calibration of 10, 15, or 20 gtt/mL.

- Microdrip sets have a calibration of 60 gtt/mL.

- The formula for calculating flow rates is

$$\frac{\text{mL/hr Volume} \times \text{Set Calibration}}{\text{Time} \,(60 \text{ min or less})}$$

- The division factor method can be used to calculate flow rates only if the volume to be administered is specified in mL/hr (60 min).

- The division factor is obtained by dividing 60 by the set calibration.

- Flow rate by the division factor method is determined by dividing the mL/hr to be administered by the division factor.

- Because microdrip sets have a calibration of 60 gtt/mL, their division factor is 1, and the flow rate in gtt/min is the same as the mL/hr ordered.

- If an IV runs ahead of or behind schedule, a possible procedure is to use the time and mL remaining to calculate a new flow rate.

- If an IV is determined to have infused ahead of schedule, immediate assessment of the individual's tolerance to the excess fluid is required and appropriate action should be taken.

- If a rate must be increased to compensate for running behind schedule, the type of fluid being infused and the individual's ability to tolerate an increased rate must be assessed.

Summary Self-Test

Answer as briefly as possible.

1. Determine the division factor for the following IV sets.

   a) 60 gtt/mL   _____

   b) 15 gtt/mL   _____

   c) 20 gtt/mL   _____

   d) 10 gtt/mL   _____

2. How is the flow rate determined in the division factor method?   _____

3. The division factor method can only be used if the volume to be
   administered is expressed in . . .   _____

4. An IV is to infuse at 50 gtt/min. How will you set it using a
   15 sec count?   _____

5. You are to adjust an IV at a rate of 60 gtt/min. What will the 15 sec
   count be?   _____

Calculate the flow rate in gtt/min.

6. An infusion of 2000 mL has been ordered to run 16 hr. The set
   calibration is 10 gtt/mL.   _____

7. The order is for 500 mL in 8 hr. The set is calibrated at 15 gtt/mL.   _____

8. Administer 150 mL in 3 hr. A microdrip is used.   _____

9. 1500 mL has been ordered to infuse in 12 hr. Set calibration
   is 20 gtt/mL.   _____

10. An IV medication of 30 mL is to be administered in 30 min using a
    15 gtt/mL set.   _____

11. Administer 100 mL in 1 hr using a 15 gtt/mL set.   _____

12. Infuse 500 mL in 6 hr. Set calibration is 10 gtt/mL.   _____

13. The order is to infuse a liter in 10 hr. At the end of 8 hr, you notice that
    there are 500 mL left. What would the new flow rate need to be to finish
    on schedule if the set calibration is 10 gtt/mL?   _____

14. An IV was started at 9 am with orders to infuse 500 mL in 6 hr.
    At noon, the IV infiltrated with 350 mL left in the bag. At 1 pm, the IV
    was restarted. The set calibration is 20 gtt/mL. Calculate the new
    flow rate to deliver the infusion on time.   _____

15. A 50 mL IV is to infuse in 15 min. The set calibration is 15 gtt/mL.
    After 5 min, the IV contains 40 mL. Calculate the flow rate to deliver
    the volume on time.   _____

16. An IV of 1000 mL is ordered to run at 25 mL/hr using a
    microdrip set.   _____

17. An infusion of 800 mL has been ordered to run in 5 hr. Set calibration
    is 10 gtt/mL.   _____

18. Administer 1500 mL in 8 hr using a set calibrated at 20 gtt/mL.   _____

19. The order is for 750 mL to run in 6 hr. Set calibration is 15 gtt/mL.   _____

20. An IV of 1000 mL was ordered to run in 8 hr. After 4 hr, only 250 mL have infused. The set calibration is 20 gtt/mL. Recalculate the rate for the remaining solution to complete on time. _____

21. The order is to infuse 50 mL in 1 hr. The set calibration is a microdrip. _____

22. An IV of 500 mL is to infuse in 6 hr using a set calibrated at 10 gtt/mL. _____

23. Infuse 120 mL in 1 hr. Set calibration is 10 gtt/mL. _____

24. Administer 12 mL in 22 min using a microdrip set. _____

25. A patient is to receive 3000 mL in 20 hr. Set is calibrated at 20 gtt/mL. _____

26. Infuse 1 liter in 5 hr using a set calibration of 15 gtt/mL. _____

27. A total of 1180 mL is to infuse in 12 hr using a set calibrated at 20 gtt/mL. _____

28. A volume of 150 mL is to infuse in 30 min. At the end of 20 min, you discover that 100 mL have infused. The set calibration is 10 gtt/mL. Should the flow rate be adjusted? If so, what is the new rate?

_____   _____

29. The order is for 1000 mL in 5 hr. The set calibration is 20 gtt/mL. _____

30. Infuse 15 mL in 14 min using a 20 gtt/mL set. _____

31. The order is for 1000 mL in 10 hr using a 20 gtt/mL calibration. _____

32. A microdrip is used to administer 12 mL in 17 min. _____

33. Infuse 2750 mL in 20 hr using a 10 gtt/mL set. _____

34. An IV of 1800 mL is to infuse in 15 hr using a 15 gtt/mL set. _____

35. Infuse 600 mL in 6 hr with a 10 gtt/mL set. _____

36. Administer 22 mL in 18 min using a mirodrip set. _____

37. An order of 1800 mL is to infuse in 10 hr. Set calibration is 20 gtt/mL. _____

38. Infuse 8 mL in 9 min using a microdrip. _____

39. Infuse 4000 mL in 20 hr. A 20 gtt/mL set is used. _____

40. An IV of 500 mL that was to infuse in 2 hr is discovered to have only 150 mL left after 30 min. Recalculate the flow rate. Set calibration is 15 gtt/mL. _____

Answers			
1. a) 1 b) 4 c) 3 d) 6	**10.** 15 gtt/min	**22.** 14 gtt/min	**33.** 23 gtt/min
2. mL/hr ÷ division factor	**11.** 25 gtt/min	**23.** 20 gtt/min	**34.** 30 gtt/min
	12. 14 gtt/min	**24.** 33 gtt/min	**35.** 17 gtt/min
3. mL/hr (mL/60 min)	**13.** 42 gtt/min	**25.** 50 gtt/min	**36.** 73 gtt/min
	14. 58 gtt/min	**26.** 50 gtt/min	**37.** 60 gtt/min
4. 13 gtt/15 sec	**15.** 60 gtt/min	**27.** 33 gtt/min	**38.** 53 gtt/min
5. 15 gtt/15 sec	**16.** 25 gtt/min	**28.** No, rate is correct at 50 gtt/min	**39.** 67 gtt/min
6. 21 gtt/min	**17.** 27 gtt/min		**40.** 25 gtt/min
7. 16 gtt/min	**18.** 63 gtt/min	**29.** 67 gtt/min	
8. 50 gtt/min	**19.** 31 gtt/min	**30.** 21 gtt/min	
9. 42 gtt/min	**20.** 63 gtt/min	**31.** 33 gtt/min	
	21. 50 gtt/min	**32.** 42 gtt/min	

CALCULATING IV INFUSION AND COMPLETION TIMES

There are a number of reasons for calculating IV infusion and completion times: to know when an IV solution will complete so that additional solutions ordered can be prepared in advance and ready to hang; to discontinue an IV when it has completed; and to label an IV bag with start, progress, and completion times so that the infusion can be monitored and adjusted to keep it on schedule. Knowing the infusion time is also important because laboratory studies are sometimes made before, during, or after specified amounts of IV solutions have infused. The infusion time may be calculated in hours and/or minutes, depending on the type and amount of solution ordered.

CALCULATING INFUSION TIME FROM mL/hr ORDERED

The infusion time is calculated for each bag/bottle to be hung and infused. The largest capacity IV solution bag or bottle is 1000 mL, but 500 mL, 250 mL, and 50 mL bags are also commonly used. Calculations for odd-numbered volumes remaining when an IV infiltrates are also routinely done. **Infusion time is calculated by dividing the volume being infused by the mL/hr rate ordered.**

Because most IVs take several hours to infuse, the unit of time being calculated most often includes hours (hr) and minutes (min).

 IV infusion time is calculated by dividing the volume to be infused by the mL/hr flow rate.

EXAMPLE 1   Calculate the infusion time for an IV of **500 mL** to infuse at **50 mL/hr.**

Infusion Time = **volume ÷ mL/hr rate**

= 500 mL ÷ 50 mL/hr = **10 hr**

The infusion time for an IV of 500 mL infusing at 50 mL/hr is 10 hr.

Objectives

The learner will calculate:

1. infusion times.

2. completion times using international/military and standard time.

3. infusion time to label IV bag/bottle with start, progress, and completion times.

EXAMPLE 2 The order is to infuse **1000 mL** at **75 mL/hr**. Calculate the infusion time.

1000 mL ÷ 75 mL/hr = **13.33 hr**

In this example, the 13 represents hr, whereas the **.33 represents the fraction of an additional hr**.

 Fractional hr are converted to min by multiplying 60 min by the fraction obtained.

Calculate min by multiplying 60 min by the fractional .33 hr.

60 min/hr × .33 hr = 19.8 = **20 min**

The infusion time is 13 hr 20 min.

EXAMPLE 3 An IV of **1000 mL** is to infuse at **90 mL/hr**. Calculate the infusion time.

1000 mL ÷ 90 mL/hr = **11.11 hr**

Remember that .11 represents the fraction of an additional hr. Convert this to min by multiplying 60 min by .11

60 min/hr × .11 hr = 6.6 = **7 min**

The infusion time is 11 hr 7 min.

EXAMPLE 4 Calculate the infusion time for **750 mL** at a rate of **80 mL/hr**.

750 mL ÷ 80 mL/hr = **9.38 hr**

60 min/hr × .38 hr = 22.8 = **23 min**

The infusion time is 9 hr 23 min.

EXAMPLE 5 A rate of **75 mL/hr** is ordered for a volume of **500 mL**. Calculate the infusion time.

500 mL ÷ 75 mL/hr = **6.67 hr**

60 min/hr × .67 hr = 40.2 = **40 min**

The infusion time is 6 hr 40 min.

Problems 17.1

Calculate the infusion times.

1. An IV of 900 mL to infuse at 80 mL/hr. _____
2. A volume of 250 mL to infuse at 30 mL/hr. _____
3. An infusion of 180 mL to run at 25 mL/hr. _____
4. A volume of 1000 mL ordered at 60 mL/hr. _____

5. An IV of 150 mL to infuse at 80 mL/hr.   _____

6. An infusion of 1000 mL at 125 mL/hr.   _____

7. A rate of 120 mL/hr for 500 mL.   _____

8. A volume of 800 mL at 60 mL/hr.   _____

9. An IV of 250 mL at 80 mL/hr.   _____

10. A rate of 135 mL/hr for 750 mL.   _____

> **Answers** **1.** 11 hr 15 min **2.** 8 hr 20 min **3.** 7 hr 12 min **4.** 16 hr 40 min **5.** 1 hr 53 min
> **6.** 8 hr **7.** 4 hr 10 min **8.** 13 hr 20 min **9.** 3 hr 8 min **10.** 5 hr 34 min
> **Note:** Answers may vary due to rounding or calculator setting, so variations of 1–2 min may be considered correct.

CALCULATING INFUSION COMPLETION TIMES

The **completion time is the actual hour and/or minute an infusion bag or bottle will complete or empty**. Completion times are calculated in either **international/ military time** using the 24-hour clock, or **standard time**, depending on individual clinical facility policy.

 The completion time is calculated by adding the infusion time to the time the IV was started.

An example is the addition of an infusion time of 90 min to a 0515 international/ military or 5:15 am standard time when an IV was started.

INTERNATIONAL/MILITARY TIME CALCULATIONS

EXAMPLE 1   An IV started at **0400** is to complete in **2 hr 30 min**. Calculate the completion time.

- **Add the 2 hr 30 min infusion time to the 0400 start time**

$$
\begin{array}{r}
0400 \\
+ \quad 230 \\
\hline
0630
\end{array}
$$

The completion time is 0630.

EXAMPLE 2   An IV started at **0750** is to complete in **5 hr 10 min**. Calculate the completion time.

- **Add the 5 hr 10 min infusion time to the 0750 start time.**

$$
\begin{array}{r}
0750 \\
+ \quad 510 \\
\hline
1260
\end{array}
$$

Change the 60 min to 1 hr and add to 1200 = 1300

The completion time is 1300.

EXAMPLE 3

An IV started at **2250** is to complete in **4 hr 20 min**. Calculate the completion time.

- **Add the infusion time to the start time.**

$$
\begin{array}{r}
2250 \\
+ \ \ 420 \\
\hline
2670
\end{array}
$$

Change the 70 min to 1 hr 10 min = 2710

Deduct 24 hr from 2710 = 0310

The completion time is 0310.

Problems 17.2

Calculate the international/military completion times.

1. An IV started at 0415 to infuse in 1 hr 30 min. _____
2. An infusion started at 1735 to complete in 2 hr 40 min. _____
3. An IV to complete in 1 hr 14 min that was started at 0025. _____
4. An IV started at 2300 to complete in 3 hr 40 min. _____
5. An infusion time of 6 hr 20 min for an infusion started at 0325. _____
6. An IV started at 0445 to complete in 3 hr 20 min. _____
7. A medication infusion started at 0740 to complete in 90 min. _____
8. An IV medication started at 1247 to complete in 45 min. _____
9. An IV started at 1430 to complete in 4 hr. _____
10. An IV started at 1605 to complete in 3 hr 30 min. _____

Answers **1.** 0545 **2.** 2015 **3.** 0139 **4.** 0240 **5.** 0945 **6.** 0805 **7.** 0910 **8.** 1332
9. 1830 **10.** 1935

STANDARD TIME CALCULATIONS

EXAMPLE 1

An IV medication will infuse in **20 minutes**. It is now **6:14 pm**. When will it complete?

- **Add the 20 minutes infusion time to the 6:14 pm start time.**

6:14 pm + **20 min** = **6:34 pm**

The completion time will be at 6:34 pm.

EXAMPLE 2

An IV is to infuse in **2 hr 33 min**. It is now **4:43 pm**. When will it complete?

- **Add the 2 hr 33 min infusion time to the 4:43 start time.**

$$
\begin{array}{r}
4:43 \text{ pm} \\
+ \ \ 2:33 \\
\hline
6:76
\end{array}
$$

Change the 76 min to 1 hr 16 min to make the completion time 7:16 pm.

The infusion will complete at 7:16 pm.

EXAMPLE 3

An IV infusion time is **13 hr 20 min.** What is its completion time if it was started at **10:45 am**?

- Add the 13 hr 20 min infusion time to the 10:45 am start time.

$$\begin{array}{r} 10{:}45 \text{ am} \\ +\ 13{:}20 \\ \hline 23{:}65 \end{array}$$

Change the 65 min to 1 hr 5 min = 24:05. Subtract 12 hr.

The completion time will be 12:05 am.

EXAMPLE 4

A IV with an infusion time of **10 hr 7 min** is started at **9:42 am.** When will it complete?

- Add the 10 hr 7 min infusion time to the 9:42 am start time.

$$\begin{array}{r} 9{:}42 \text{ am} \\ +\ 10{:}07 \\ \hline 19{:}49 \end{array}$$

Subtract 12 hr to make the completion time 7:49 pm.

The completion time will be 7:49 pm.

EXAMPLE 5

An IV with an infusion time of **12 hr 30 min** is started at **2:10 am.** When will it complete?

- Add the 12 hr 30 min infusion time to the 2:10 am start time.

$$\begin{array}{r} 2{:}10 \text{ am} \\ +\ 12{:}30 \\ \hline 14{:}40 \end{array}$$

Subtract 12 hr to make the time 2:40 pm.

The completion time will be 2:40 pm.

Problems 17.3

Calculate IV completion using standard time.

1. An IV started at 4:40 am that has an infusion time of 9 hr 42 min. _____

2. An IV medication started at 7:30 am that has an infusion time of 45 min. _____

3. An IV with an infusion time of 7 hr 7 min that was restarted at 10:42 am. _____

4. An IV with a restart time of 9:07 pm has an infusion time of 6 hr 27 min. _____

5. An IV with an infusion time of 3 hr 30 min was started at 11:49 pm. _____

6. An IV started at 2:43 pm to infuse in 40 min. _____

7. An IV medication started at 10:15 am to complete in 90 min. _____

8. An infusion started at 7:05 pm to complete in 8 hr. _____

9. An IV started at 5:47 am to complete in 5 hr. _____

10. An IV started at 4:20 am to complete in 12 hr. _____

> **Answers 1.** 2:22 pm **2.** 8:15 am **3.** 5:49 pm **4.** 3:34 am **5.** 3:19 am **6.** 3:23 pm **7.** 11:45 am
> **8.** 3:05 am **9.** 10:47 am **10.** 4:20 pm

LABELING SOLUTION BAGS WITH INFUSION AND COMPLETION TIMES

IV bags/bottles are calibrated so that the amount of fluid remaining can be checked at any time. In the majority of clinical facilities it is routine to label bags when they are hung with start, progress, and finish times to provide a visual reference of the status of the infusion. Commercially prepared labels are available for this purpose; however, you can prepare one using any tape available.

Refer to Figure 17-1, where you can see closeup the calibrations on a 1000 mL bag. Notice that each 50 mL is calibrated but that only the 100 mL calibrations are numbered: 1, 2, 3 (for 100, 200, 300), etc. Also, notice that the calibrations on the IV bag are not all the same width. They are somewhat wider at the bottom because gravity and the pressure of the solution force more fluid to the bottom of the bag.

The tape on the IV solution bag in Figure 17-1 is for an 8 hr infusion, from 9 am to 5 pm. The 9A represents the start time of 9 am, and the 5P at the bottom represents the completion time of 5 pm. An 8 hr infusion time for 1000 mL means that 125 mL are to be infused per hour (1000 mL ÷ 8 hr = 125 mL/hr). Each 125 mL is labeled on the calibrated scale along with the hour the IV should be at this level. This tape allows for constant visual

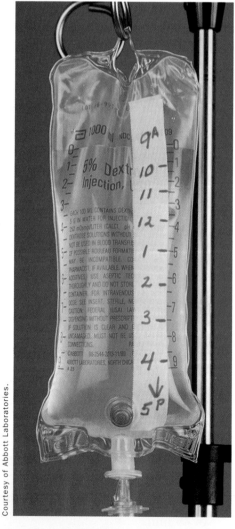

Courtesy of Abbott Laboratories.

Figure 17-1

monitoring of the IV. Regardless of your clinical responsibility, develop the habit of reading infusion time labeling, particularly if you have been giving personal care that involves movement or repositioning of the patient.

Let's look at an example of how you could label an IV that is just being started.

EXAMPLE 1   An IV of **1000 mL** has been ordered to run at **150 mL/hr**. It was started at **1:40 pm** Tape the bag with start, progress, and completion times.

Add the tape to the bag/bottle so that it is near but does not cover the calibrations. Enter the start time as 1:40 pm at the 1000 mL level. Next, mark each 150 mL from top to bottom with the successive hours the IV will run.

1000 mL − 150 mL = 850 mL	Label 850 mL for 2:40 pm
850 mL − 150 mL = 700 mL	Label 700 mL for 3:40 pm
700 mL − 150 mL = 550 mL	Label 550 mL for 4:40 pm
550 mL − 150 mL = 400 mL	Label 400 mL for 5:40 pm
400 mL − 150 mL = 250 mL	Label 250 mL for 6:40 pm
250 mL − 150 mL = 100 mL	Label 100 mL for 7:40 pm

Calculate the infusion time for the remaining 100 mL.

$$100 \text{ mL} \div 150 \text{ mL/hr} = 0.66 = \textbf{0.67 hr}$$

$$60 \text{ min/hr} \times 0.67 \text{ hr} = 40.2 = \textbf{40 min}$$

$$7{:}40 \text{ pm} + \textbf{40 min} = \textbf{8:20 pm}$$

The completion time is 8:20 pm.

EXAMPLE 2   An infiltrated IV with **625 mL** remaining is restarted at **5:30 pm** to run at **150 mL/hr**. Relabel the bag with the new start, progress, and completion times.

Label the 625 mL level with the 5:30 pm restart time.

625 mL − 150 mL = 475 mL	Label 475 mL for 6:30 pm
475 mL − 150 mL = 325 mL	Label 325 mL for 7:30 pm
325 mL − 150 mL = 175 mL	Label 175 mL for 8:30 pm
175 mL − 150 mL = 25 mL	Label 25 mL for 9:30 pm

Calculate the infusion time for the remaining 25 mL.

$$25 \text{ mL} \div 150 \text{ mL/hr} = 0.166 = \textbf{0.17 hr}$$

$$60 \text{ min/hr} \times 0.17 \text{ hr} = 10.2 = \textbf{10 min}$$

$$9{:}30 \text{ pm} + \textbf{10 min} = \textbf{9:40 pm}$$

The completion time is 9:40 pm.

EXAMPLE 3   An infiltrated IV with **340 mL** remaining is restarted at **4:15 am** to run at **70 mL/hr**. Relabel the bag with the new start, progress, and completion times.

Label the 340 mL level with the 4:15 am restart time.

340 mL − 70 mL = 270 mL	Label 270 mL for 5:15 am
270 mL − 70 mL = 200 mL	Label 200 mL for 6:15 am
200 mL − 70 mL = 130 mL	Label 130 mL for 7:15 am
130 mL − 70 mL = 60 mL	Label 60 mL for 8:15 am

Calculate the infusion time for the remaining 60 mL.

60 mL ÷ 70 mL/hr = 0.857 = **0.86 hr**

60 min/hr × 0.86 hr = 51.6 = **52 min**

8:15 am + **52 min** = **9:07 am**

The completion time is 9:07 am.

Problems 17.4

Calculate the infusion and completion times. Label the IV bags provided with start, progress, and completion times. Have your instructor check your labeling.

1. The IV in Figure 17-2 of 1000 mL was started at 0710 to run at 75 mL/hr.

    Infusion time _____   Completion time _____

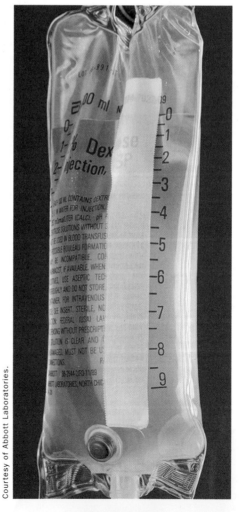

Courtesy of Abbott Laboratories.

Figure 17-2

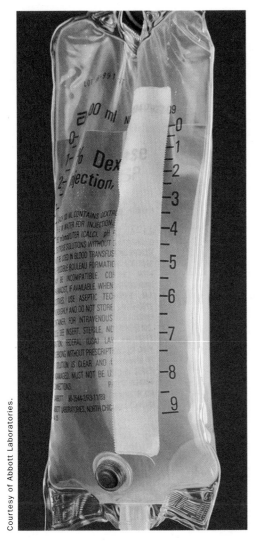

Courtesy of Abbott Laboratories.

Figure 17-3

Courtesy of Abbott Laboratories.

Figure 17-4

2. The 1000 mL IV in Figure 17-3 has an ordered rate of 125 mL/hr. It was started at 6:30 pm.

Infusion time _____   Completion time _____

3. The IV in Figure 17-4 of 1000 mL has an ordered rate of 80 mL/hr. It was started at 5:40 am.

Infusion time _____   Completion time _____

Answers   **1.** 13 hr 20 min; 2030   **2.** 8 hr; 2:30 am   **3.** 12 hr 30 min; 6.10 pm

Summary

This concludes the chapter on calculation of infusion and completion times and labeling of IV bags/bottles with start, progress, and completion times. The important points to remember from this chapter are:

- The infusion time is the time required for an IV to infuse completely.

- The infusion time is calculated by dividing the total volume to infuse by the mL/hr rate ordered.

- The completion time is calculated by adding the infusion time to the start time.

- When the min calculated are 60 or more, an additional hr is added to the completion time and 60 min are subtracted from the total min.

- Calculating completion times provides an opportunity to plan ahead and have the next solution ordered ready to hang or to discontinue an IV when it has completed.

- Most clinical facilities label IV solution bags/bottles with start, progress, and finish times to provide a visual record of the infusion status.

Summary Self-Test

Calculate the infusion and completion times.

1. The order is for 50 mL to infuse at 50 mL/hr. The infusion was started at 10:10 am.

   Infusion time _____   Completion time _____

2. An infusion of 950 mL is ordered at 80 mL/hr. It was started at 8:02 am.

   Infusion time _____   Completion time _____

3. A total of 280 mL remain in an IV bag. The flow rate is 70 mL/hr. It is now 11:03 am.

   Infusion time _____   Completion time _____

4. The order is to infuse 500 mL at 90 mL/hr. The IV was started at 2:40 pm.

   Infusion time _____   Completion time _____

5. An infiltrated IV with 850 mL remaining is restarted at 10 am at a rate of 150 mL/hr.

   Infusion time _____   Completion time _____

6. At 4:04 am, an IV of 500 mL is started at a rate of 50 mL/hr.

   Infusion time _____   Completion time _____

7. An IV medication with a volume of 150 mL is started at 1:45 pm to infuse at 60 mL/hr.

   Infusion time _____   Completion time _____

8. An IV of 520 mL is restarted at 0420 at a rate of 125 mL/hr.

   Infusion time _____   Completion time _____

9. It is 12:00 pm, and an IV of 900 mL is to infuse at a rate of 100 mL/hr.

   Infusion time _____   Completion time _____

10. An IV of 1000 mL is started at 0550 to infuse at 130 mL/hr.

    Infusion time _____   Completion time _____

11. An infusion of 250 mL is started at 11:20 am to infuse at a rate of 20 mL/hr.

    Infusion time _____   Completion time _____

12. The flow rate ordered for 1 L is 80 mL/hr. It was started at 8:07 pm.

    Infusion time _____   Completion time _____

13. A 250 mL volume is started at 3:40 pm to be infused at 90 mL/hr.

Infusion time _____   Completion time _____

14. A medication volume of 100 mL is started at 4:00 pm to infuse at 42 mL/hr.

Infusion time _____   Completion time _____

15. At 11:00 pm, 200 mL remain in an IV. The rate is 120 mL/hr.

Infusion time _____   Completion time _____

16. An infusion of 350 mL is to run at 150 mL/hr. It is now 9:47 am.

Infusion time _____   Completion time _____

17. An IV medication of 25 mL is started at 8:17 am to run at 25 mL/hr.

Infusion time _____   Completion time _____

18. An IV of 425 mL is restarted at 0814 to infuse at 90 mL/hr.

Infusion time _____   Completion time _____

19. At 10:30 pm, there are 180 mL left in an IV that is infusing at 25 mL/hr.

Infusion time _____   Completion time _____

20. At 1400, 500 mL is started to run at a rate of 60 mL/hr.

Infusion time _____   Completion time _____

21. An infusion of 250 mL is started at 3:04 am to run at 100 mL/hr.

Infusion time _____   Completion time _____

22. With 525 mL remaining, a rate change to 108 mL/hr is ordered. It is 2:10 am.

Infusion time _____   Completion time _____

23. A liter is started at 8:42 am at a rate of 120 mL/hr.

Infusion time _____   Completion time _____

24. An infusion of 1000 mL is to run at 200 mL/hr. It is started at 6:40 pm.

Infusion time _____   Completion time _____

25. An IV medication of 100 mL is started at 7:50 am to run at 150 mL/hr.

Infusion time _____   Completion time _____

26. A volume of 500 mL is started at 4:04 pm at a rate of 75 mL/hr.

Infusion time _____   Completion time _____

27. An IV of 950 mL is restarted at 2:10 am at 100 mL/hr.

Infusion time _____   Completion time _____

28. An IV medication of 30 mL is started at 0915 at a rate of 60 mL/hr.

Infusion time _____   Completion time _____

29. A medication volume of 90 mL was started at 6:15 am to be infused at 90 mL/hr.

Infusion time _____   Completion time _____

30. A rate of 80 mL/hr is set at 4:20 pm to infuse a medication with a volume of 100 mL.

Infusion time _____   Completion time _____

31. A volume of 750 mL is started at 0303 at a rate of 96 mL/hr.

Infusion time _____   Completion time _____

Label the following solution bags for the times and rates indicated. Have your instructor check your labeling.

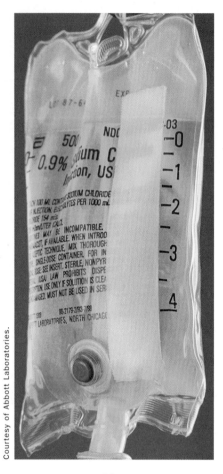

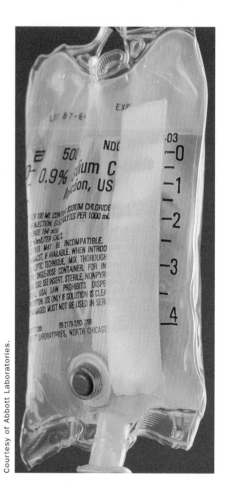

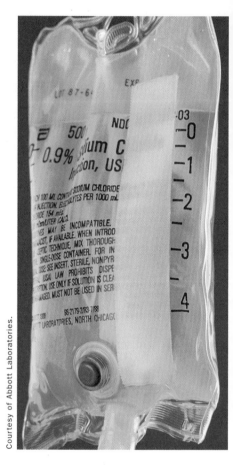

32.
Started: 10:47 am
Rate: 80 mL/hr

33.
Started: 1315
Rate: 100 mL/hr

34.
Started: 2:10 pm
Rate: 90 mL/hr

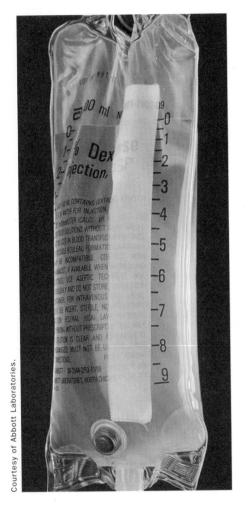

Courtesy of Abbott Laboratories.

35.
Started: 0440
Rate: 75 mL/hr

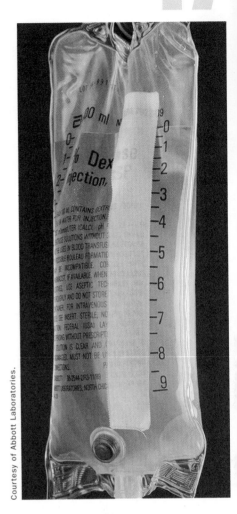

Courtesy of Abbott Laboratories.

36.
Started: 0730
Rate: 50 mL/hr

Courtesy of Abbott Laboratories.

37.
Started: 6:20 pm
Rate: 25 mL/hr

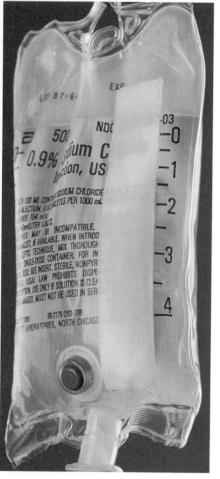

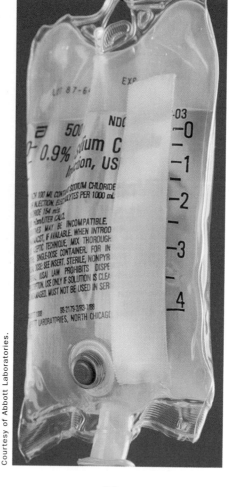

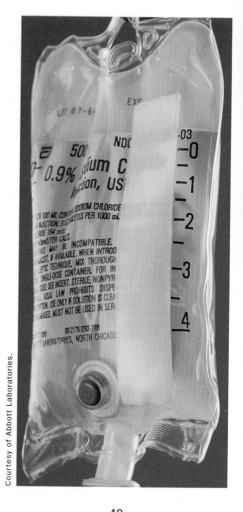

38.
Started: 3:03 am
Rate: 50 mL/hr

39.
Started: 0744
Rate: 125 mL/hr

40.
Started: 2140
Rate: 100 mL/hr

Answers

1. 1 hr; 11:10 am
2. 11 hr 53 min; 7:55 pm
3. 4 hr; 3:03 pm
4. 5 hr 34 min; 8:14 pm
5. 5 hr 40 min; 3:40 pm
6. 10 hr; 2:04 pm
7. 2 hr 30 min; 4:15 pm
8. 4 hr 10 min; 0830
9. 9 hr; 9 pm
10. 7 hr 41 min; 1331

11. 12 hr 30 min; 11:50 pm
12. 12 hr 30 min; 8:37 am
13. 2 hr 47 min; 6:27 pm
14. 2 hr 23 min; 6:23 pm
15. 1 hr 40 min; 12:40 am
16. 2 hr 20 min; 12:07 pm
17. 1 hr; 9:17 am
18. 4 hr 43 min; 1257
19. 7 hr 12 min; 5:42 am
20. 8 hr 20 min; 2220
21. 2 hr 30 min; 5:34 am

22. 4 hr 52 min; 7:02 am
23. 8 hr 20 min; 5:02 pm
24. 5 hr; 11:40 pm
25. 40 min; 8:30 am
26. 6 hr 40 min; 10:44 pm
27. 9 hr 30 min; 11:40 am
28. 30 min; 0945
29. 1 hr; 7:15 am
30. 1 hr 15 min; 5:35 pm
31. 7 hr 49 min; 1052
32-40. Verify your answers with your instructor.

Note: Answers may vary slightly due to rounding.

HEPARIN INFUSION CALCULATIONS

Objectives

The learner will calculate:

1. heparin dosages.

2. mL/hr flow rates for an EID.

3. hourly dosage infusing from mL/hr rate.

Heparin is a powerful anticoagulant drug that inhibits new blood clot formation, or the extension of already-existing clots. Heparin is commonly mixed in IV solutions for administration, especially postoperatively to prevent clot fomation from venous stasis. Heparin IV use is so frequent that it is prepared in ready-to-hang IV bags, such as the **1000 units (2 units/mL) strength illustrated** in Figure 19-1. Notice on this bag that **heparin and its dosage strength is clearly printed in red**, as a safety factor to distinguish it from other intravenous solutions.

Heparin can also be administered subcutaneously in small dosages. Subcutaneous injections require **deep injection at a 45° angle** to discourage bleeding from medication leaking through the injection tract. Also, **subcutaneous sites are not massaged after injection**, again to prevent bleeding at the site.

Heparin dosages may be based on body weight in kg, or on a patient's clotting time. Because of heparin's potent anticoagulant action, clotting times are checked frequently during administration.

There is no essential difference in the calculations you have already practiced for critical care dosages and those for heparin dosages, except that heparin dosages for subcutaneous injection are measured using a TB syringe. However, heparin's action is so critical that it does deserve to be addressed separately. In this chapter, you will be introduced to labels of a variety of heparin dosages, practice measuring heparin dosages for addition to IV solutions, calculate units per hour infusing from mL/hr flow rates, and be reminded of the precautions used to maintain patency of intravenous injection ports.

HEPARIN IV AND VIAL LABELS

Let's start by taking a look at the heparin IV solution bag in Figure 19-1. This is an example of premixed IV solution. Notice the blue "Heparin Sodium 1,000 units in 0.9% Sodium Chloride Injection" labeling on this 500 mL bag and the red dosage labeling "Heparin 1,000 units (2 units/mL)" printed sideways on the top right. The red dosages draw particular attention to

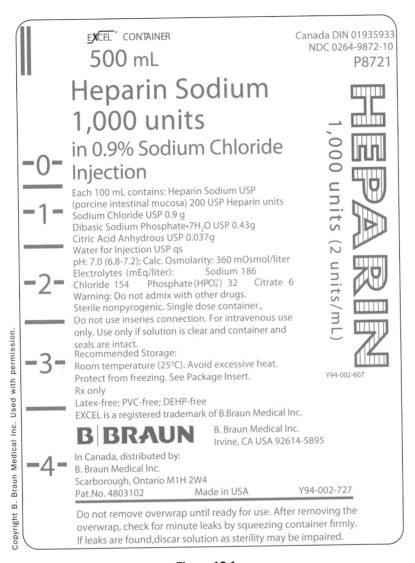

Figure 19-1

the fact that these bags contain heparin, and make the bags instantly recognizable. They serve as an important safety factor in solution identification.

If a commercially prepared IV heparin dosage strength that you require is not available, you may be required to prepare the solution yourself from **a number of available vial dosage strengths**. Let's stop and look at the vial labels in Figures 19-2 through 19-5, so that you can refresh your memory with some typical calculations.

Problems 19.1

Read the heparin labels provided to determine how many mL of heparin will be necessary to prepare the solutions indicated.

1. Refer to the label in Figure 19-2 to determine how many mL will be required to add 20,000 units to an IV solution. _____

2. Refer to the label in Figure 19-3 to determine how many mL will be required to add 20,000 units to an IV solution. _____

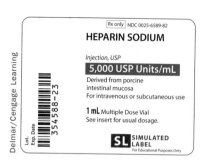

Figure 19-2

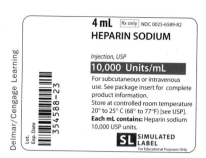

Figure 19-3

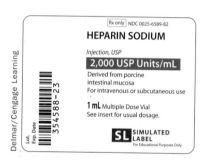

Figure 19-4

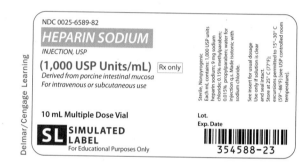

Figure 19-5

3. Refer to the label in Figure 19-4 to determine how many mL of heparin will be required to add 12,000 units to an IV solution. _____

4. Refer to the label in Figure 19-5 to determine how many mL will be required to add 10,000 units to an IV solution. _____

Answers   **1.** 4 mL   **2.** 2 mL   **3.** 6 mL   **4.** 10 mL

CALCULATING mL/hr IV FLOW RATE FROM units/hr ORDERED

Because heparin is most frequently ordered in units/hr to be administered—for example, 1000 units/hr—and infused using an EID (electronic infusion device), a common calculation will be for the mL/hr flow rate needed for this dosage. Let's look at these calculations first, keeping in mind that **the mL/hr flow rate for an EID is identical to the gtt/min rate for a microdrip.**

EXAMPLE 1   The order is to infuse heparin **1000 units/hr** from a solution of **20,000 units in 500 mL** D5W. Calculate the **mL/hr** flow rate.

Enter the mL/hr being calculated first. Locate the ratio containing mL, the 20,000 units/500 mL strength, and enter this as the starting ratio with mL as the numerator, to match the mL numerator of the units being calculated; 20,000 units becomes the denominator.

$$\frac{mL}{hr} = \frac{500 \ mL}{20,000 \ units}$$

The starting ratio denominator, units, must be matched in the next numerator. Enter the 1000 units/hr rate ordered, with units as the numerator. This completes the equation.

$$\frac{mL}{hr} = \frac{500 \text{ mL}}{20{,}000 \text{ units}} \times \frac{1000 \text{ units}}{1 \text{ hr}}$$

Cancel alternate denominator/numerator units in the equation to double-check that the ratios have been entered correctly. Only mL and hr should remain. Do the math.

$$\frac{mL}{hr} = \frac{500 \text{ mL}}{20{,}000 \text{ units}} \times \frac{1000 \text{ units}}{1 \text{ hr}} = 25 \text{ mL/hr}$$

A rate of 25 mL/hr is required to infuse 1000 units/hr from a solution strength of 20,000 units in 500 mL.

EXAMPLE 2   The order is for heparin **800 units/hr**. The solution available is **40,000 units in 1000 mL D5W**. Calculate the **mL/hr** flow rate.

Enter the mL/hr being calculated. Enter the 1000 mL/40,000 units ratio, with mL as the numerator.

$$\frac{mL}{hr} = \frac{1000 \text{ mL}}{40{,}000 \text{ units}}$$

Enter the next ratio, 800 units/hr, with 800 units as the numerator to match the starting ratio denominator.

$$\frac{mL}{hr} = \frac{1000 \text{ mL}}{40{,}000 \text{ units}} \times \frac{800 \text{ units}}{1 \text{ hr}}$$

Cancel to double-check for correct ratio entry, and do the math.

$$\frac{mL}{hr} = \frac{1000 \text{ mL}}{40{,}000 \text{ units}} \times \frac{800 \text{ units}}{1 \text{ hr}} = 20 \text{ mL/hr}$$

A rate of 20 mL/hr is required to infuse 800 units/hr from a solution strength of 40,000 units in 1000 mL.

EXAMPLE 3   The order is to infuse heparin **1100 units/hr** from a solution strength of **60,000 units in 1 L D5W**. Calculate the **mL/hr** flow rate.

$$\frac{mL}{hr} = \frac{1000 \text{ mL}}{60{,}000 \text{ units}} \times \frac{1100 \text{ units}}{1 \text{ hr}}$$

$$\frac{mL}{hr} = \frac{1000 \text{ mL}}{60{,}000 \text{ units}} \times \frac{1100 \text{ units}}{1 \text{ hr}} = 18.33 = 18 \text{ mL/hr}$$

A rate of 18 mL/hr will be required to infuse 1100 units per hour from a 60,000 units in 1 L solution.

Problems 19.2

Calculate the mL/hr flow rates.

1. The order is to infuse 1000 units heparin per hour from an available solution strength of 25,000 units in 500 mL D5W. _____

2. Heparin has been ordered at 2500 units per hour. The solution strength is 50,000 units in 1000 mL D5W. _____

3. The order is to infuse 1100 units per hour from a 15,000 units in 1 L D5W solution. _____

4. An adult has orders for 50,000 units of heparin in 1000 mL D5W to infuse at a rate of 2000 units per hour. _____

5. Administer 1500 units per hour of heparin from an available strength of 40,000 units in 1 L. _____

Answers **1.** 20 mL/hr **2.** 50 mL/hr **3.** 73 mL/hr **4.** 40 mL/hr **5.** 38 mL/hr

CALCULATING units/hr INFUSING FROM mL/hr FLOW RATE

On occasion it may be necessary to calculate the units/hr of heparin infusing from the mL/hr flow rate. This is done using the units/mL solution strength and mL/hr rate of infusion.

EXAMPLE 1 An IV of **1000 mL** containing **40,000 units** of heparin is running at **30 mL/hr**. Calculate the **units/hr** infusing.

$$\frac{\text{units}}{\text{hr}} = \frac{40,000 \, \text{units}}{1000 \, \text{mL}} \times \frac{30 \, \text{mL}}{1 \, \text{hr}}$$

$$\frac{\text{units}}{\text{hr}} = \frac{40,000 \, \text{units}}{1000 \, \text{mL}} \times \frac{30 \, \text{mL}}{1 \, \text{hr}} = \textbf{1200 units/hr}$$

A 1000 mL solution containing 40,000 units heparin running at 30 mL/hr is infusing 1200 units/hr.

EXAMPLE 2 A solution of **1 L** of D5W with **20,000 units** heparin is running at **80 mL/hr**. Calculate the **units/hr** infusing.

$$\frac{\text{units}}{\text{hr}} = \frac{20,000 \, \text{units}}{1000 \, \text{mL}} \times \frac{80 \, \text{mL}}{1 \, \text{hr}}$$

$$\frac{\text{units}}{\text{hr}} = \frac{20,000 \, \text{units}}{1000 \, \text{mL}} \times \frac{80 \, \text{mL}}{1 \, \text{hr}} = \textbf{1600 units/hr}$$

A 1 L (1000 mL) solution containing 20,000 units heparin running at 80 mL/hr is infusing 1600 units/hr.

EXAMPLE 3   An IV of D5W **500 mL** containing **10,000 units** heparin is running at **40 mL/hr**. Calculate the **units/hr** infusing.

$$\frac{\text{units}}{\text{hr}} = \frac{10{,}000 \text{ units}}{500 \text{ mL}} \times \frac{40 \text{ mL}}{1 \text{ hr}}$$

$$\frac{\text{units}}{\text{hr}} = \frac{10{,}000 \text{ units}}{500 \text{ mL}} \times \frac{40 \text{ mL}}{1 \text{ hr}} = \textbf{800 units/hr}$$

A 500 mL solution containing 10,000 units heparin running at 40 mL/hr is infusing 800 units/hr.

Problems 19.3

Calculate the units/hr of heparin infusing in the IV administrations.

1. An IV of 750 mL containing 30,000 units heparin running at 25 mL/hr.   _____

2. A solution of 20,000 units in 500 mL running at 30 mL/hr.   _____

3. A 1 L volume of D5W containing heparin 30,000 units running at 40 mL/hr.   _____

4. An IV of 1 L DNS containing 20,000 units heparin running at 30 mL/hr.   _____

5. A 25,000 units heparin in 500 mL solution running at 30 mL/hr.   _____

6. An IV of 1000 mL containing 40,000 units heparin running at 25 mL/hr.   _____

7. A 1000 mL solution with 45,000 units heparin running at 25 mL/hr.   _____

8. A solution of 1000 mL containing 25,000 units heparin running at 30 mL/hr.   _____

9. A 1 L solution with 35,000 units heparin running at 45 mL/hr.   _____

10. A 20,000 units in 500 mL solution running at 20 mL/hr.   _____

Answers   1. 1000 units/hr   **2.** 1200 units/hr   **3.** 1200 units/hr   **4.** 600 units/hr   **5.** 1500 units/hr
6. 1000 units/hr   **7.** 1125 units/hr   **8.** 750 units/hr   **9.** 1575 units/hr   **10.** 800 units/hr

HEPARIN FLUSH DOSAGE

As you learned in an earlier chapter, heparin flush solutions used to maintain patent (open) indwelling IV infusion ports come in **two dosage strengths: 10 units/mL and 100 units/mL.**

You have just learned that **heparin vial dosage strengths available for IV dilution range from 1,000 to 50,000 units/mL.** So it is time now to be reminded of the **enormous difference in dosage strengths between the 10 to 100 units/mL flush solutions, and the 1,000 to 50,000 units/mL intravenous admixture dosage strengths.**

Misreading heparin labels can be life-threatening. Too large a dosage used for a flush will cause systemic hemorrhage; too small a dosage added to an IV can lead to death from venous stasis and clot emboli.

 The average IV port heparin flush dosage is 10 units, and never exceeds 100 units.

Summary

This concludes the chapter on heparin administration. The important points to remember are:

- Heparin is a potent anticoagulant that is frequently added to IV solutions.

- It is measured in USP units.

- Heparin therapy requires a frequent check of coagulation times.

- Subcutaneous heparin injections are given deep subcutaneously at a 45° angle in an attempt to reduce medication leakage through the injection track.

- Heparin injection sites are never massaged.

- IV heparin may be ordered by mL/hr flow rate or by units/hr to infuse.

- An EID or microdrip is used for heparin infusion.

- Commercially prepared IV heparin solutions are available in several strengths.

- Additional IV solution strengths may require the preparation of heparin from available 1000 to 50,000 units/mL vial strengths.

- Frequent blood tests for clotting time are required to monitor heparin dosage.

- Heparin IV port flushes never exceed 100 units.

Summary Self-Test

Calculate the mL/hr heparin flow rates.

1. An adult is to receive heparin 1000 units/hr. The IV solution available has 25,000 units in 1 L D5W, and a pump will be used. _____

2. A solution of 35,000 units heparin in 1 L D5W is to infuse via volumetric pump at 1200 units/hr. _____

3. The order is for 1000 units heparin per hour. The solution strength is 20,000 units in 500 mL D5NS. _____

4. The order is for 1250 units/hr heparin from a solution strength of 15,000 units in 500 mL D5W. A pump is used to monitor the infusion. _____

5. A solution of 10,000 units heparin in 500 mL D5W is ordered to infuse at 1000 units/hr. _____

6. An IV of 1000 mL D5W with 40,000 units heparin is to infuse at
   1200 units/hr via a pump.   _____

7. The order is to infuse 500 mL D5W with 25,000 units heparin at
   1500 units/hr.   _____

8. 500 mL D5W with 30,000 units of heparin is to infuse via a pump at
   1500 units/hr.   _____

9. The order is to infuse 1 L D5W with 45,000 units of heparin at 1875 units/hr.   _____

10. A rate of 500 units/hr is ordered using a 250 mL with 10,000 units
    IV solution.   _____

11. A solution of 40,000 units in 1000 mL is to be used to infuse 1500 units/hr.   _____

12. A rate of 1500 units/hr is ordered using a 30,000 units in 500 mL solution.   _____

13. Heparin 750 units/hr is ordered using an IV solution of 500 mL containing
    5000 units heparin.   _____

14. An IV solution of 10,000 units in 1000 mL heparin is to infuse 500 units/hr.   _____

15. Heparin 1500 units per hour is to be infused using a solution strength of
    15,000 units in 500 mL.   _____

Answers

1. 40 mL/hr
2. 34 mL/hr
3. 25 mL/hr
4. 41.6 or 42 mL/hr
5. 50 mL/hr

6. 30 mL/hr
7. 30 mL/hr
8. 25 mL/hr
9. 41.6 or 42 mL/hr
10. 12.5 or 13 mL/hr
11. 37.5 or 38 mL/hr

12. 25 mL/hr
13. 75 mL/hr
14. 50 mL/hr
15. 50 mL/hr

Equivalents

Metric Equivalents	Household Equivalents	Approximate Equivalents
1 g = 1,000 mg = 1,000,000 mcg	3 t = 1 T	1 t = 5 mL
0.001 g = **1 mg** = 1,000 mcg	2 T = 1 fl oz	1 T = 3 t = 15 mL = $\frac{1}{2}$ fl oz
0.000001 g = 0.001 mg = **1 mcg**	1 cup = 8 fl oz	1 fl oz = 30 mL = 6 t
1 kg = 1,000 g	1 pt = 16 fl oz = 2 cups	1 L = 1 qt = 32 fl oz = 2 pt = 4 cups
1 L = 1,000 mL	1 qt = 2 pt = 4 cups = 32 fl oz	1 pt = 16 fl oz = 2 cups
0.001 L = **1 mL**	1 lb = 16 oz	1 cup = 8 fl oz = 240 mL
1 m = 100 cm = 1,000 mm		1 kg = 2.2 lb
0.01 m = **1 cm** = 10 mm		1 in = 2.5 cm
0.001 m = 0.1 cm = **1 mm**		

Rounding Decimals

For many dosage calculations, it will be necessary to compute decimal calculations to *thousandths* (*three* decimal places) and round back to *hundredths* (*two* places) for the final answer. For example, pediatric care and critical care require this degree of accuracy. At other times, you will need to round to *tenths* (*one* place). Let's look closely at this important math skill.

RULE

To round a decimal to hundredths, drop the number in thousandths place, and

1. Do not change the number in hundredths place if the number in thousandths place was 4 or less.

2. Increase the number in hundredths place by 1 if the number in thousandths place was 5 or more.

When rounding for dosage calculations, unnecessary zeros can be dropped. For example, 5.20 rounded to hundredths place should be written as 5.2, because the 0 is not needed to clarify the number.

EXAMPLES ■

Tenths	Hundredths	Thousandths	
			All rounded to hundredths (2 places)

0 . 1 2 3   = 0.12

1 . 7 4 4   = 1.74

5 . 3 2 5   = 5.33

0 . 6 6 6   = 0.67

0 . 3 0   = 0.3   (When this is rounded to hundredths, the final zero should be dropped. It is not needed to clarify the number and is potentially confusing.)

RULE

To round a decimal to tenths, drop the number in hundredths place, and

1. Do not change the number in tenths place if the number in hundredths place was 4 or less.

2. Increase the number in tenths place by 1 if the number in hundredths place was 5 or more.

EXAMPLES ■

Tenths	Hundredths	
		All rounded to tenths (1 place)

0 . 1 3   = 0.1

5 . 6 4   = 5.6

0 . 7 5   = 0.8

1 . 6 6   = 1.7

0 . 9 5   = 1.0 = 1   (The zero at the end of this decimal number is dropped, because it is unnecessary and potentially confusing.)